SYNAPZ
The Complete Final MBBS Manual: Format Book

Editors

McEnroe D Mordom MBBS
Government Medical College
Calicut, Kerala, India

Mridulal A MBBS
Government Medical College
Calicut, Kerala, India

Randeep AM MBBS
Government Medical College
Calicut, Kerala, India

JAYPEE *The Health Sciences Publisher*

New Delhi | London | Philadelphia | Panama

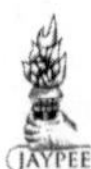

Jaypee Brothers Medical Publishers (P) Ltd.

Headquarters
Jaypee Brothers Medical Publishers (P) Ltd.
4838/24, Ansari Road, Daryaganj
New Delhi 110 002, India
Phone: +91-11-43574357
Fax: +91-11-43574314
E-mail: jaypee@jaypeebrothers.com

Overseas Offices

J.P. Medical Ltd.
83, Victoria Street, London
SW1H 0HW (UK)
Phone: +44-20 3170 8910
Fax: +44(0)20 3008 6180
E-mail: info@jpmedpub.com

Jaypee-Highlights Medical Publishers Inc.
City of Knowledge, Bld. 237, Clayton
Panama City, Panama
Phone: +1 507-301-0496
Fax: +1 507-301-0499
E-mail: cservice@jphmedical.com

Jaypee Medical Inc.
The Bourse
111, South Independence Mall East
Suite 835, Philadelphia, PA 19106, USA
Phone: +1 267-519-9789
E-mail: jpmed.us@gmail.com

Jaypee Brothers Medical Publishers (P) Ltd.
17/1-B, Babar Road, Block-B, Shaymali
Mohammadpur, Dhaka-1207
Bangladesh
Mobile: +08801912003485
E-mail: jaypeedhaka@gmail.com

Jaypee Brothers Medical Publishers (P) Ltd.
Bhotahity, Kathmandu, Nepal
Phone: +977-9741283608
E-mail: kathmandu@jaypeebrothers.com

Website: www.jaypeebrothers.com
Website: www.jaypeedigital.com

Inquiries for bulk sales may be solicited at: jaypee@jaypeebrothers.com

SYNAPZ—The Complete Final MBBS Manual: Format Book

First Edition: 2008

Second Edition: **2015**

ISBN: 978-93-5152-890-6

Printed at Rajkamal Electric Press, Plot No. 2, Phase-IV, Kundli, Haryana.

Dedicated to

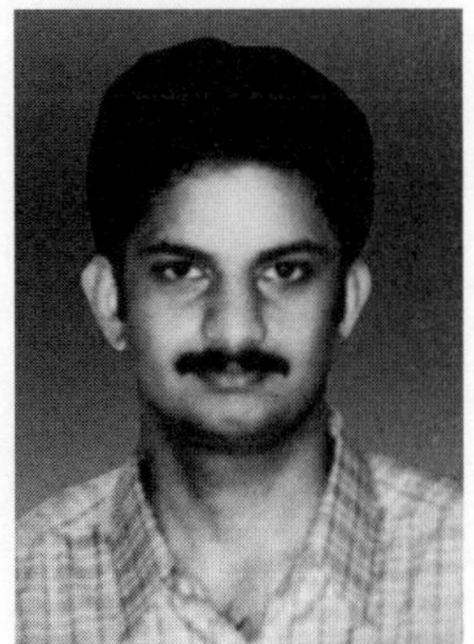

Late Dr Saju P

On a fateful January 26th, 2001 he embarked on a journey with a noble cause as a part of National Service Scheme-Mathrubhumi medical team to provide relief to the earthquake stricken people of Gujarat, India. On February 2nd, putting duty before life, he left this world serving humanity to his last breath; his soul shines eternally as a guiding light for everyone...............

Contributors

MEDICINE

Mukund A Prabhu
Alumni, Government Medical College
Calicut, Kerala, India

P Sandeep
Alumni, Government Medical College
Calicut, Kerala, India

SURGERY

Sreejith Nair
Alumni, Government Medical College
Calicut, Kerala, India

Jayan
Alumni, Government Medical College
Calicut, Kerala, India

ORTHOPEDICS

Rejith Valsalan
Alumni, Government Medical College
Calicut, Kerala, India

C Anoop
Alumni, Government Medical College
Calicut, Kerala, India

Nikhil
Alumni, Government Medical College
Calicut, Kerala, India

OBSTETRICS AND GYNECOLOGY

Anjali Prem
Alumni, Government Medical College
Calicut, Kerala, India

Geovin Ranji
Alumni, Government Medical College
Calicut, Kerala, India

PEDIATRICS

Arun Abhilash
Alumni, Government Medical College
Calicut, Kerala, India

Preface to the Second Edition

It is our pleasure to introduce the second edition of *SYNAPZ—The Complete Final MBBS Manual: Format Book.* This book is designed to provide a concise summary of subjects taught in your final year MBBS. In the second edition, the entire book has been revised, with a view to eliminating errors, incorporating suggestions of readers, updating concepts, and discarding material that is no longer relevant. In this way, the book has been kept concise while remaining as up-to-date and accurate as possible. In keeping with the current trend of postgraduate entrance examinations, all topics are updated. Key points and comparisons are given in boxes for greater emphasis.

In shaping and revising this latest edition, we have committed ourselves to making the manual an invaluable resource for students.

We have revised the outline format used in last edition hoping to organize information in a logical and readily accessible format. In our quest to polish the second edition of the manual, we have sought to retain the virtues that have made the work a success. Each session has case-taking format followed by concise discussion of relevant topics. Alongside format modifications, we have carefully updated the contents of the manual to reflect advancing medicine. We added a section for objective structured clinical examination (OSCE), hoping it will be useful in exam preparation. We hope you will be benefited by the chest X-ray section with basics in chest radiology. We hope the collection of frequently asked questions will make your exam preparation easy. Operative procedures are briefly narrated for rapid recollection. Mnemonics sections are elaborated and definitions are added at end of sections in view of students' special interest.

We are greatly indebted to the many individuals who helped with the preparation of the book. Those who have really helpful in preparation of this edition including Dr Mukund A Prabhu, Dr Aquil Kalanad, Dr Sreejith Nair, Dr Jayan, Dr Rejith Valsalan, Dr Anjali Prem, Dr Geovin Ranji and Dr Arun Abhilash.

The book will not be complete without mention of the Students, Interns, Residents and Teachers of Calicut Medical College. We are inspired daily by their brilliance, compassion and dedication.

We thank our families for their support and inspiration.

Finally, we would like to thank M/s Jaypee Brothers Medical Publishers (P) Ltd., New Delhi, India, for giving us this greatest opportunity.

McEnroe D Mordom
Mridulal A
Randeep AM

Preface to the First Edition

SYNAPZ is an attempt of academic cooperation and self-help.

We know that final MBBS examination is too hard a nut to crack for an average medical student who does not have adequate dexterity familiarity with the examination pattern and frequently asked questions. It is obvious that along with a thorough theoretical knowledge, we need a sufficiently tactical approach based on common sense, which is an essential prerequisite for a sure success in the examinations especially for the practical sessions.

SYNAPZ is envisaged as a simple epistemological tool capable of bringing about a delightful compromise between the vast academic curriculum and the strictly constrained time period to tackle it. This is not supposed to replace the textbook, but can be used as a tool for effective exploration of the syllabus with a sense of sequential importance.

SYNAPZ consists of a collection of frequently asked questions, case format for all subjects, case discussion, mnemonics, practical examination tips, objective structured clinical examination (OSCE), diagram, surgical procedure and normal values.

McEnroe D Mordom
Mridulal A

Acknowledgments

Our heartfelt gratitude to Dr C Raveendran, Principal, Government Medical College, Calicut; Dr PK Sasidharan, Professor and Head, Department of General Medicine, Government Medical College, Calicut; Dr MP Sasi, Professor and Head, Department of Surgery, Government Medical College, Calicut; Dr Jyodish, Professor and Head, Department of Orthopedics, Government Medical College, Calicut; Dr Umadevi, Professor and Head, Department of Obstetrics and Gynecology, Government Medical College, Calicut; Dr Khadeeja Mumthaz, Professor, Department of Obstetrics and Gynecology, Government Medical College, Calicut; Dr Riyas A, Professor and Head, Department of Pediatrics, Government Medical College, Calicut; Dr Balraj G, Associate Professor, Department of Pediatrics, Government Medical College, Calicut; Dr Johnson Marion, Department of ENT, Nirmala Hospital, Calicut; Dr Premu Vensor, Consultant Gynecologist, Asian Reproductive Medicine Centre (ARMC), Calicut; Dr A Shibulal, SCTIMST, Thiruvananthapuram; Dr Seena S Lal, Assistant Professor, Department of Physiology, Government Medical College, Thrissur; Dr Bishara M Lal, Department of Physiology, Medical College, Thrissur; Dr Akhil Pushkar, Alumni, Amrita Institute of Medical Sciences, Kochi; Dr Lal Antony and Dr Shreeja Lal, Alumni, Medical College, Calicut; Dr Madhusudanan ES, Department of Anesthesiology, Government Medical College, Thrissur; Dr Ashok SK, Alumni, Government Medical College, Calicut; Dr Rohan Raj, Alumni, Government Medical College, Calicut; Dr Unniraja, Alumni, Government Medical College, Calicut; Dr Ushabhayi C, Department of Pharmacology, Academy of Medical Sciences, Pariyaram; Dr Nabil A and Dr Jinu Annie Jose, Alumni, Government Medical College, Calicut; Dr Firoz Khan V and Dr Fathima, Alumni, Government Medical College, Calicut; Dr Nishanth MN, Alumni, Government Medical College, Calicut; Dr Namitha, Alumni, Academy of Medical Sciences, Pariyaram; Dr Prasoon Thomas Joseph and Dr Sayooj KM, Alumni, Government Medical College, Calicut; Dr Mithun S and Dr Minu S, Alumni, Government Medical College, Calicut; Dr Keerthi Mohan, Alumni, Amrita Institute of Medical Sciences, Kochi; Dr Pramod R Pillai, Alumni, Amrita Institute of Medical Sciences, Kochi; Dr Nisha Kumari, Alumni, Amrita Institute of Medical Sciences, Kochi; Dr Deepa Dinesh, Alumni, Amrita Institute of Medical Sciences, Kochi; Dr Emil Joseph Eliston, Alumni, Amrita Institute of Medical Sciences, Kochi; Dr Arjun Krishnan, Alumni, Amrita Institute of Medical Sciences, Kochi; Dr P Raju and Dr Lakshmi, Alumni, Government Medical College, Calicut; Dr U Faizal and Dr Noufira, Alumni, Medical College, Calicut; Dr Mahesh Kumar D and Dr Khayas EK, Alumni, Government Medical College, Calicut; Dr Manoj Kumar E and Dr Vijun, Alumni, Government Medical College, Calicut; Dr Jithesh AK and Dr Suneesh Kumar K, Alumni, Government Medical College, Calicut; Dr Praveen TM and Dr Rimsy P, Alumni, Government Medical College, Calicut; Dr Jyothish Hari and Dr Anup Ahmed, Alumni, Government Medical College, Calicut; Dr Shabeerali K and Dr Abdusammad T, Alumni, Government Medical College, Calicut; Dr Aneesh George and Dr Anish Mohan, Alumni, Government Medical College, Calicut; Dr Mithun Vasudevan and Dr Febin P, Alumni, Government Medical College, Calicut; Dr Wales T George, Alumni, Government Medical College, Calicut; Dr Aslam Farooq ZA and Amjad Farooq ZA, Alumni, Government Medical College, Calicut; Dr Byju P, Alumni, Government Medical College, Calicut; Dr Jayesh Narayanan and Dr Anas N, Alumni, Government Medical College, Calicut; Dr Alex M and Dr Badira, Alumni, Government Medical College, Calicut; Dr Anish KP and Dr Anugunu, Alumni, Government Medical College, Calicut; Dr Sreehari GK, Alumni, Government Medical College, Calicut; Dr Sameeha Saidalavi, Alumni, Government Medical College, Calicut; Dr Santhosh Kumar N and Dr Jimil Francis, Alumni, Government Medical College, Calicut; Dr Vivek Raju, Alumni, Government Medical College, Calicut; Dr Sreekanth P and Dr Rohini, Alumni, Government Medical College, Calicut; Dr Aneesh KP, Alumni, Government Medical College, Calicut; Dr Rahul Raveendran, Alumni, Medical College, Calicut; Dr Anish KA and Dr Mathews Vergese Maret, Alumni, Government Medical College, Calicut; Dr Abdu Raheem Kapoor and Dr Sarath MB, Alumni, Government Medical College, Calicut; Dr Abhilash B and Dr Divya CK, Alumni, Government Medical College, Calicut; Dr Subheesh P, Alumni, Government Medical College, Calicut; Dr Thamizharasi A, General Duty Medical Officer, PHC, Thirubhuvanai, Puducherry; Dr Davidson Devasia, Alumni, Jubilee Mission Medical College, Thrissur; Dr Manjunath PS, Alumni, Jubilee Mission Medical College, Thrissur, Dr Abin Sooraj, Alumni, MES Medical College, Perinthalmanna; Dr Percy Mathew, Alumni, Amala Medical College, Thrissur; Dr Rahees Abdulla, Alumni, Amala Medical College, Thrissur; Dr Anoob PT and Dr Praveen, Government Medical College, Calicut; Mr Praveen Raj and Rani, Alumni, College of Pharmaceutical Sciences,

Calicut; Benita Francis and Felina Francis, MBBS Students, Gokulam Medical College, Trivandrum, Kerala, India.

We acknowledge our sincere gratitude to our parents, teachers and also to 44th (2000) and 48th (2004) Batch MBBS Government Medical College, Calicut, Kerala, India.

We thank to Balesh and Sandeep, Associates, Government Medical College, Calicut; Mr Selvaraj PS, Artist, Department of Anatomy, Government Medical College, Calicut; Raju PG, 50th Batch MBBS Student, Government Medical College, Calicut; Anand Krishnan, Nithin Akkal, Navaneeth SB, Rajesh IR, 52nd Batch MBBS Students, Medical College, Calicut; Mr Niyesh, "Samagra", Calicut; Mr Sanoj, "Printers Fort", Calicut; Adv Shijo, Legal Advisor, Calicut; CAMPUS PULSE, Government Medical College, Calicut, Kerala, India.

Contents

1 Medicine

GENERAL EXAMINATION

Pallor

- Ensure adequate lighting
- Evert lower eyelids
- Other areas—tongue, hard palate, nail beds, palms, palmar crease
- Most common cause of anemia—hookworm.

Pallor without Anemia

- Myxedema
- Vasovagal attack
- Nephritic syndrome
- Peripheral circulatory failure.

Icterus

- Ensure adequate natural daylight, do not use a torch
- Examine both posterior sclera when patient looks down
- Other areas—soft palate, palms, skin.

Cyanosis

- Ensure adequate lighting
- Examine over tongue, oral mucosa, lips
- Other areas—cheeks, ear lobes, tip of nose, hands, nail beds.

Sites in Peripheral Cyanosis

- Tip of the nose
- Ear lobules
- Outer aspect of lips, chin and cheek
- Tip of the fingers and toes
- Palms and soles
- Tongue remains unaffected.

Sites to be Looked for in Central Cyanosis

- Tongue (mainly the margin as well as the under surface)
- Inner aspect of lips
- Mucous membrane of gum, soft palate, cheeks
- Lower palpebral conjunctiva
- Plus, the sites mentioned in the peripheral cyanosis.

Clubbing

- Examine the finger nails tangentially or do Shamroth's sign
- Palpate the nail bed for fluctuation
- Look for widening and tenderness of end of long bones—hypertrophic osteoarthropathy.

Grading of Clubbing

Grade 1: Obliteration of the angle between nail and nail bed and positive fluctuation test.
Grade 2: Parrot beak appearance.
Grade 3: Drumstick appearance.
Grade 4: Hypertrophic osteoarthropathy.

Types of Clubbing

- Drum stick—congenital cyanotic heart disease and bronchiectasis
- Parrot beak—bronchogenic carcinoma
- Painful clubbing—bronchogenic carcinoma and SBE
- Unilateral—presubclavian coarctation of aorta, bronchogenic carcinoma, cervical rib, aneurysm of subclavian artery, erythromelalgia, arteriovenous fistula of branchial vessels
- Unidigital—hereditary, local trauma, sarcoidosis, rarely from median nerve injury or deposition of tophi
- Pseudoclubbing—scleroderma, acromegaly, hyperthyroidism and leprosy.

Lymphadenopathy

Lymph Nodes in Cervicofacial Area

- Make the patient sit comfortably
- Approach the patient from behind
- Flex the patient's neck forward

- Ask the patient to incline his neck to the side of examination
- Palpate lymph node from the same side
- Examine the occipital, posterior auricular, preauricular, submandibular, submental, superficial and deep cervical lymph nodes, lymph nodes in posterior triangle
- Examine both sides.
  [**Comment on:** Location, size, shape, tenderness, number, texture, fixity].

Lymph Nodes in the Axilla

- Approach the patient from front
- Insert the right hand into the patient's left axilla
- Patient's arm is adducted and his forearm rests comfortably on examiner's forearm
- Make the patients opposite shoulder steady
- Slide the finger against the chest wall
- Palpate the anterior axillary fold
- Palpate the lateral axillary wall (using left hand for the left side palm directed laterally against the upper end of humerus)
- Palpate the posterior axillary fold from behind
- Examine both sides.

Epitrochlear Nodes

- Make patients elbow semiflexed
- Place your right palm over the posterior aspect of the patient's right elbow and vice versa
- The epitrochlear lymph nodes (LNs) can now be palpated under your thumb
- Move the thumb in anteroposterior direction for better appreciation
- Other LNs to be palpated—inguinal, abdominal, popliteal.

Edema

- Use your thumb for applying firm pressure for 5 to 30 seconds behind the medial malleolus of tibia
- Other sites—over sacrum, abdominal wall, malar bones
- Examine both sides
  [**Comment:** Unilateral or bilateral; pitting or nonpitting; sites involved].

If the dimple fills within 40 seconds indicates **hypoproteinemia**. If it takes more than 40 seconds indicates **cardiac failure**.

Causes of Pitting Edema

- Congestive cardiac failure
- Cirrhosis of liver
- Nephrotic syndrome
- Hypoproteinemia with severe anemia
- Pericardial effusion
- Constrictive pericarditis
- Drugs—nifedipine, liquorice, corticosteroid, estrogen
- Venous obstruction
- Beriberi, epidemic dropsy.

Causes of Nonpitting Edema

- Myxedema
- Lymphatic edema
- Angioneurotic edema
- Scleroderma (poststreptococcal, self-limited, painless edematous induration).

Evolution of Edema in Different Systemic Diseases

- *Congestive cardiac failure:* Legs—face—ascites
- *Nephrotic syndrome:* Face (periorbital puffiness)—legs—ascites
- *Cirrhosis of liver:* Ascites—legs—face
- *Nutritional edema:* Edema feet with puffiness of face—ascites.

VITALS

Arterial Pulse

- *Radial pulse:* Semipronated forearm; flex the wrist feel the pulse near the wrist and examine it for a minute.
- *Carotid pulse:* Ask the patient to look straight ahead use your thumb and press it backwards at the level of medial border of sternomastoid muscle and lateral to thyroid cartilage. Character of the pulse is best felt.

- *Popliteal pulse:* Ask the patient to lie supine make knee partially flexed feel pulse with fingers encircling and supporting the knee from both sides.
- *Posterior tibial pulse:* Ask the patient to lie supine and feel the pulse in the groove midway between medial malleolus and the heel (tendo-Achilles).
- *Dorsalis pedis pulse*: Feel the pulse lateral to the extensor hallucis longus tendon and proximal to first metatarsal space. Examine both sides simultaneously except carotid pulse.
  [**Comment:** Rate, rhythm, character, volume, condition of vessel wall, other peripheral pulses, radiofemoral delay, radioradial delay].

Causes of relative bradycardia
- Any viral fever
- First week of enteric fever
- Sometimes in pyogenic meningitis
- Brucellosis, psittacosis.

Causes of relative tachycardia
- Acute rheumatic carditis
- Tuberculosis
- Diphtheritic myocarditis
- Polyarteritis nodosa.

Respiratory Rate and Rhythm

- Put the patient at ease
- Place the palm lightly on abdominal wall or chest
- Keep an eye on the watch; count the rate for a minute.
  [**Comment on:** Rate, rhythm (regular/irregular), character and depth].

Temperature

- Dip the thermometer in an antiseptic and wipe dry
- Shake down the mercury column below the normal temperature
- Explain the procedure to the patient
- Keep the thermometer sublingually
- Patient's lips are firmly closed
- Keep it in place for at least a minute
- Take readings immediately holding horizontally
- Other sites—rectal, axillary, groin.

Temperature Ranges

	Centigrade	Fahrenheit
Normal	36.6–37.2	98–99
Subnormal	< 36.6	<98
Febrile	>37.2	>99
Hyperpyrexia	>41.6	>107
Hypothermia	<35	>95

JUGULAR VENOUS PULSE AND PRESSURE

- Patient is reclined at 45° at hip
- The neck is supported to relax the muscles
- Face turned to left
- Use good lighting
- View tangentially the internal jugular vein
- Time with opposite carotid pulse or apex
- Measure the vertical height using 2 scales with the sternal angle as reference point.
  [**Comment on:** Height (in centimeter above the sternal angle) and waveform (a, c, v, x, y)].

CARDIOVASCULAR SYSTEM

Presenting Complaints

- Breathlessness on exertion/at rest (Orthopnea, PND)
- **Palpitation:** 1. Fast/slow; 2. Regular/irregular; 3. At rest/exertion; 4. If at rest emotional or not.
- Central chest pain
- Cough
- Sputum (color, quantity, smell)
- Hemoptysis
- Pedal edema
- Syncope.

Examination of CVS

Example of how to report:

- **Pulse**—72 per minute, regular, normal in volume, and character, no brachiofemoral delay, no radioradial delay. All the peripheral pulses felt normally on both sides. Vessel wall not thickened. (No pulse deficit, if pulse is irregular).

- **Blood pressure** is 120/80 mm Hg in the right upper limb in the supine position. (a) Patient not on any antihypertensives. (b) If on antihypertensives take BP in both sitting/lying down and standing position).
- **Jugular venous pressure** is 5 cm above the sternal angle. Hepato-jugular reflux present.

Inspection

- Shape of precordium (and look for any skeletal deformities)
- Apical impulse seen/not seen; if seen where?
- Other pulsations (suprasternal, epigastrium, back, parasternal)
- Engorged veins on the chest wall
- Any other findings mention if present (like scars, sinus, accessory nipple).

Palpation

- Apex beat—Location, character, thrills if any (Comment on the position only in the supine, sitting or leaning forward. In case the apex beat is still not felt look in the left lateral position, but comment only on the character and thrill and not on the position).
- Palpability of heart sounds (for example, palpable P2 in pulmonary hypertension).
- Left parasternal heave.
- Thrills if any in all areas.
- Any other pulsations (epigastric, suprasternal).

Percussion

- Liver dullness
- Right border of heart
- Left border of heart—dullness starts at the apex
- Second left intercostal space.

Auscultation

Look for the following in all the auscultatory areas:

- First and second HS
- Additional sounds (IIIrd and IVth HS)
- Any murmurs

- Adventitious sounds (click, rub)
- Pericardial rub if present.

N.B.: In case of cardiomegaly, do not mention the apex as the mitral area, name it as the apex. The auscultatory areas are fixed. All auscultatory areas may be mentioned with respect to the apex and the intercostal spaces to avoid confusion. Neoaortic (Erbs area) is the 3rd left intercostal area near the sternal border. The EDM of AR is best heard here.

Other systems (relevant findings to look for)

- Basal creps for pulmonary edema
- Hepatomegaly, ascites and pedal edema for right heart failure
- Splenomegaly and other signs of IE
- Signs of neurological deficits (due to embolism).

Diagnosis

This is a case of mitral stenosis probably due to rheumatic heart disease. There are no signs of congestive cardiac failure. No features of rheumatic reactivation and of infective endocarditis and the patient is in sinus rhythm at present. Effort intolerance grade (mention the grade).

Mitral Stenosis

Low pitched rough rumbling mid-diastolic murmur with presystolic accentuation of grade III intensity heard best in the mitral area without any radiation with the bell of the stethoscope with the patient lying in the left lateral position and the breath held in expiration. Intensity of the murmur increases with mild exercise.

Mitral Regurgitation

High pitched soft blowing pansystolic murmur of grade IV intensity heard best in the mitral area radiating to the left axilla and inferior angle of scapula heard best with the diaphragm of the stethoscope with the patient lying in the left lateral position and the breath held in expiration.

Aortic Stenosis

High pitched harsh ejection systolic murmur of grade V intensity heard best in the aortic area radiating to the carotids best heard with the diaphragm of the stethoscope with the patient sitting up and leaning forward with the breath held in expiration.

Aortic Regurgitation

High pitched soft blowing. Early diastolic murmur of grade III intensity heard best in the neoaortic area with the diaphragm of the stethoscope with the patient sitting up and leaning forward with the breath held in expiration.

Auscultatory Areas

- Mitral—5th left ICS 1 cm medial to MCL
- Tricuspid—lower part of sternum
- Aortic—2nd right ICS at the sternal margin
- Pulmonary—2nd left ICS at the sternal margin
- Neoaortic area—3rd left ICS at the sternal margin
- Apex (if cardiomegaly+).

Examination Tips

Inspection of the Precordium

- Expose the chest wall well
- Patient lies supine or sits if orthopneic
- Look for precordial bulge tangentially (from the foot end of the patient or from the sides)
- Locate the apex beat.
  [**Comment on:** Precordial pulsations—suprasternal, sternal, aortic area, parasternal area, epigastrium].

Thoracic cage abnormality—kyphosis, scoliosis, pectus excavatum, pectus carinatum, emphysema.

Palpation of Apical Area

- Expose the precordium well
- Ask the patient to lie supine or sit if orthopneic
- Localize the apex beat by inspection
- Use ulnar border of the right hand to palpate the apex
- Further localize the apex with the tip of index finger
- Put the patient in left lateral position to assess the character of apex better.

Murmur 10 Points

1. Site
2. Pitch
3. Timing
4. Grade

5. Character
6. Radiation
7. Positional variation
8. Variation with respiration
9. Best heard with bell/diaphragm
10. Variation with exercise/exertion.
    [**Comment:** Site of the apex beat; character (normal, hyperdynamic, heaving, tapping); palpable sounds and thrills at apex].

Percussion of the Heart

- Expose the precordium well
- Ask the patient to sit or stand with his palms placed over the head
- Hold the pleximeter parallel to the cardiac border
- Percuss from resonant to dull area
- Define the left cardiac border (3rd, 4th and 5th spaces)
- Define right cardiac border
- Define the dullness of cardiac and pulmonary areas.

Auscultation of Apex

- Expose the patient adequately
- Ask the patient to lie supine
- Ensure adequate lighting
- Always time with carotid pulse to avoid confusion between systolic and diastolic events
- Localize the apex.

RESPIRATORY SYSTEM

Presenting Complaints

- Cough
- Sputum
- Hemoptysis
- Lateral chest pain
- Breathlessness
- Wheezing.

Examination of Respiratory System

Respiratory rate is 18 per minute, regular, normal in depth, abdomino-thoracic in type, patient not dyspneic.

Visible Part of Upper Respiratory Tract

- Nasal cavity (polyps, DNS, discharge)
- Paranasal sinus tenderness
- Posterior pharyngeal wall
- Postnasal discharge
- Tonsils
- Ear discharge.

Inspection

- Nasal alae moving or not
- Position of trachea
- Shape of the chest
  - Hollowing
  - Kyphoscoliosis
  - Flattening
  - Pectus carinatum
  - Drooping
  - Pectus excavatum
- Spine
- Apical impulse
- Movement of chest
- Intercostal suction
- Accessory muscle movement
- Wheeze/stridor
- Venous prominence.

Palpation

- Position of trachea—tracheal tug, movement and displacement
- Movements of the chest (In 3 areas apex from behind, anteriorly and posteriorly)
- Chest expansion in cms + hemithorax
- Tactile vocal fremitus in all lung fields
- Other palpable findings (e.g. rattling).

Percussion

- Start with direct percussion over the clavicle
- Normal resonance is obtained in all the lung fields on both sides

- Liver dullness is felt in the 5th right ICS in the MCL
- Tidal percussion
- Traube's space +/–
  Krönig's isthmus
- Coin percussion in pneumothorax.

Lung Fields

- Supraclavicular (above clavicle)
- Infraclavicular (clavicle to 3rd rib)
- Mammary (3rd to 6th rib)
- Inframammary (below 6th rib only on left side)
- Axillary (above 4th rib in MAL)
- Infra-axillary (below 4th rib in MAL)
- Suprascapular
- Interscapular.

Auscultation

- Breath sounds—intensity and character
- Adventitious sounds continuous or otherwise
- Crepitations—Inspiratory or expiratory; coarse or fine.

Rhonchi

- Inspiratory or expiratory
- Mono or polyphonic:
  - Vocal resonance (just mention whether equal, increased or decreased)
  - Pleural rub present/not.

Diagnosis

Hydropneumothorax

- Horizontal upper fluid level
- Shifting dullness
- Succusion splash
- Coin sound.

Percussion Notes

- *Tympanic:* Stomach/cheek
- *Hyperresonant:* Pneumothorax

- *Resonant:* Normal
- *Impaired*: Consolidation
- *Dull:* Consolidation
- *Stony dull:* Pleural effusion.

In Suspected Malignancy of the Lung Specially Look for

- SVC obstruction
- Gynecomastia
- Myopathy
- Troisier's sign
- Cerebellar sign
- Horner's syndrome
- Acanthosis nigricans
- Cushingoid features
- Hypertrophic pulmonary—osteoarthropathy.

Examination Tips

Position of Trachea

- Fix the head and place the patients chin in neutral position
- Examine from the front
- Comment on the trail's sign (sternomastoid sign) whether the clavicular head of sternomastoid is unduly prominent on one side
- Gently thrust the index or middle finger into the suprasternal notch exactly in the midline and try to feel both sides of the trachea.

Palpation of Respiratory Movements

- Grip the sides of the chest wall with the fingers
- Actively stretched thumbs should meet in the midline
- Ensure that there is a loose fold of skin between the two thumbs
- Ask the patient to take deep breaths
- At apex of lung appreciate up and down movements
- At mammary areas appreciate horizontal movements
- At infrascapular areas appreciate horizontal movements
- For apex of lung examine from front; behind and in supine position.

Chest Measurements

- Ask the patient to take deep breath and exhale fully
- Measure at the level of 4th ICS (nipples).

[**Comment on:** (a) chest expansion in cm; (b) dimensions of each hemithorax; (c) anteroposterior and transverse diameters (use 2 scales kept on chest wall appropriately); (d) Spinoscapular distance].

Examination of Vocal Fremitus

- Patient repeats one, one or ninety nine, ninety nine
- Use ulnar border of the hand
- Palpate all areas sequentially
- Immediately compare the corresponding area of the opposite side.
  [**Comment on:** (a) normal/abnormal; (b) whether increased, decreased or absent VF].

Percussion of the Lungs

Apical regions

- Tap directly on the most prominent part of the clavicle (direct percussion)
- Percuss in both supraclavicular fossae
- Define the resonance of Kronig's isthmus
- Compare the resonance on both sides.

Basal regions

- Percuss interscapular areas
- Percuss infrascapular areas
- Percuss infra-axillary areas
- Compare on both sides at each level
- Define lower border of lung anteriorly, laterally and posteriorly middle lobe regions (right) or lingular lobe region (left)
- Percuss anteriorly in 4th and 5th intercostal spaces
- Compare both sides.

Liver dullness

Tidal percussion.

Auscultation of Lungs

- Ask the patient to sit or stand
- Ask the patient to take deep regular breaths through his mouth auscultate all areas of the lungs (anteriorly, laterally and posteriorly)
- Compare both sides.
  [**Comment on:** Intensity of breath sound (normal, increased, decreased) character of breathing—vesicular, bronchial (tubular, cavernous, amphoric) or bronchovesicular; adventitious sounds—wheezes, crackles, pleural rub].

Examination of Vocal Resonance

- Ask the patient to say one repeatedly
- Auscultate all areas sequentially
- Immediately compare the corresponding area of the opposite side. [**Comment** as normal, increased, decreased VR **Comment on** bronchophony, whispering pectoriloquy or egophony].

Tracheal Tug

- Raise the chin of the patient in the midline
- Approach from the front of the patient
- Apply firm upward pressure on the two sides of the cricoid cartilage (using 1 or both sides)
- Feel for a downward tug with each heartbeat.

Succussion Splash

- Ask the patient to sit
- Stabilize the opposite shoulder
- Vigorously shake the ipsilateral shoulder
- Auscultate on the same side for succussion splash.

GASTROINTESTINAL SYSTEM

Cardinal Symptoms

- Anorexia, nausea and vomiting
- Dysphagia to solids/liquids
- Jaundice
- Pain abdomen
- Hematemesis/melena
- Diarrhea/constipation
- Alteration in bowel habit
- Abdominal distension/edema
- Oliguria/hematuria
- Neuropsychiatric manifestation in a case of liver disease.

Examination of the Gastrointestinal System

Oral Cavity

- Lips
- Teeth
- Gums, cheek and palate

- Tongue
- Fauces and tonsils
- Breath.

Inspection
- Shape and movement of the abdomen
- Distended or not
- Position and shape of umbilicus
- Dilated veins if any
- Any visible swelling/peristalsis
- Condition of skin (striae, scar, etc.)
- Hernial orifice and external genitalia.

Palpation
- Temperature
- Tenderness
- Any mass
- Pulsations
- Direction of flow of engorged veins
- Liver and gallbladder
- Spleen
- Kidney (renal angle tenderness)
- Hernial orifice and external genitalia.

Liver

______ cm palpable below the costal margin in the right MCL
- Moving with respiration
- Tender/not
- Consistency—firm/soft/hard
- Surface—smooth/irregular
- Border—sharp/rounded
- Left lobe palpable or not
- Pulsatile or not
- Palpable bruit present or not.

Percussion
- General note of the abdomen
- Upper border of liver
- Shifting dullness
- Fluid thrill
- Puddle sign if minimal fluid
- Tidal percussion.

Auscultation

- Peristaltic sounds
- Hepatic/splenic rub
- Venous hum
- Bruit.

(Remember to evacuate the patient's bladder before examining the abdomen).

Examination Tips

Palpation of the Liver

- Ask the patient to lie supine with the abdomen well-exposed
- Ask the patient to flex both his hips and knees
- Ask the patient to relax the abdominal wall
- Begin palpating from the right iliac fossa
- Keep the index finger parallel to the rib margin
- Mould the hand over the abdominal wall
- Proceed upwards till liver border is felt.

  [**Comment on:** Size, margins, surface, consistency, tenderness moving with respiration and pulsations of liver].

Span of Liver by Percussion

- Determine the upper border of the liver by heavy percussion
- Percuss down along each interspace and onto the abdomen until the liver dullness disappears
- Mark the lower border of the liver
- Measure the distance between the upper and lower border in the right midclavicular line.

Palpation of Spleen

- Ask the patient to lie supine with the abdomen relaxed
- Ask the patient to flex both hips and knees
- Ask the patient to relax the abdominal wall (quiet breathing)
- Begin examining from right iliac fossa
- Proceed towards the left hypochondrium
- Turn the patient to right lateral position for detection of early splenic enlargement.

  [**Comment on:** Size (enlarged along the axis of spleen below the costal margin in the left midclavicular line), consistency, surface and tenderness of the spleen, moving with respiration].

Bimanual method: Along with the above maneuvers using the left hand, exert gentle pressure from the posterior aspect of the left costal margin to push the abdominal contents forwards.

Dipping method (in case of ascites): The speed of dipping fingers is so important that floating organs do not have time to drift away.

- Stand on the left side of the patient. Place the hand on the lower chest and hook the fingers around the costal margin while the patient breathes deeply.

Engorged Veins over the Abdominal Wall

- Ask the patient to stand up
- Expose the abdominal wall
- Choose a length of vein without a tributary
- Using 2 fingers, milk out the vein for 3 to 4 cm
- Observe the speed of filling in either direction
- Auscultate using the bell placed highly for the presence of a venous hum.

  [**Comment on:** The site, pattern, direction of flow, probable etiology].

Percussion of Spleen

- Ask the patient to lie in right lateral position
- Percuss over the posterolateral wall of the abdominal cavity (especially around the 9th, 10th and 11th ribs)
- Determine the area of splenic dullness.

Puddles Sign (Puddle-Small Fluid Collection)

- Ask the patient to lie in the prone position for about 5 minutes
- Patient goes into the knee-elbow or knee wrist position (so that the middle portion of the abdomen is most dependent)
- Percuss the most dependent part of the abdomen for dullness
- Percuss nearby nondependent parts to compare the resonance
- Change the patient's position
- Repercussion to demonstrate resonance in the area which was previously dull.

Shifting Dullness

- Ask the patient to lie supine
- Start percussion in the epigastrium
- Continue along the midline till dullness is obtained or till the umbilicus is reached

- Percuss laterally from the most resonant point in the midline
- Define the dullness level in both flanks
- Keep the pleximeter on dull area to one side and turn the patient to the opposite side
- Wait for about 10 to 30 seconds
- Repercuss to demonstrate resonance in the area which was previously dull
- Examine on both sides.

Fluid Thrill

- Ask the patient to lie supine
- Ask the patient or his attendant (bystander) to place the ulnar border of his palm in the midline
- Gently tap on one side
- Perceive thrill on the opposite side.

CENTRAL NERVOUS SYSTEM

Cardinal Symptoms

(Always mention the onset of each symptom whether abrupt or insidious).

Higher Functions

- Abnormal consciousness
- Abnormalities of speech
- Seizures.

Cranial Nerves

Abnormalities of speech, visual disturbances, diplopia, squint, drooping of eyelid, numbness, tingling over face, difficulty in mastication, deviation of angle of mouth, inability to close eye, hyperacusis, drooling of saliva, loss of taste, hearing loss, vertigo, tinnitus, nasal regurgitation, nasal twang, dysphagia, dysarthria, hoarseness of voice.

Motor System

- Weakness
  - Upper limb
    - Proximal—raising hands
    - Distal—buttoning and unbuttoning

- Lower limb
    - Proximal—standing up from squatting or sitting
    - Distal—slipping of footwears
- Involuntary movements, wasting fasciculations
- Clumsiness of movements
- Swaying to one side, other gait abnormalities (if any).

Sensory System

- Numbness, its distribution
- Paresthesia—tingling, pins and needle sensation. Its distribution, Hyperesthesia (e.g. Thalamic syndrome)
- Root pain
- Girdle like sensation.

Autonomic Functions

- Incontinence of urine
- Retention of urine
- Hesitancy, urgency
- Bowel incontinence
- Postural giddiness/hypotension.

Raised ICT

- Vomiting (projectile)
- Headache
- Diplopia.

Others

Fever, weight loss, arthritis, rash (also in hemiplegia—ask for history of chest pain, breathlessness and palpitation).

Examination of Nervous System

Higher Functions (COMISH)

- *Consciousness:* If unconscious mention the grading.
- Orientation in time, place and person
- Memory—recent and past
- Intelligence
- Speech (test for fluency, comprehension, naming, repetition, reading and writing)
- Handedness (also look for primitive reflexes) (mention handedness in history itself).

Cranial Nerves (CN)

	Right	*Left*
1. Ist CN	N	N
2. IInd CN		
• Visual acuity	N	N
• Visual field	N	N
• Color vision	N	N
3. III, IV, VIth CN		
• No ptosis, squint or diplopia		
• Ocular movements in six cardinal positions of gaze	Full	Full
• Pupil - Size	N	N
- Shape	N	N
- Position	Central	Central
• Reflexes		
Direct light reflex	N	N
Consensual light reflex	N	N
Accommodation reflex	N	N
4. Vth CN		
Sensory		
• Touch, pain, temperature over face (test 3 divisions separately)	N	N
• Conjunctival and corneal reflexes.	N	N
Motor		
• Position of jaw on opening mouth	N	N
• Temporalis and masseter (prominence on clenching teeth)	N	N
• Jaw jerk	N	N
5. VIth CN		
• Wrinkling of forehead	N	N
• Closing of eyes	N	N
• Nasolabial fold	N	N
• Angle of mouth on showing teeth	N	N
• Whistling	N	N
• Blowing	N	N
• Platysma	N	N
• Hyperacusis	Absent	Absent
• Taste on anterior 2/3 of tongue	N	N
6. VIIIth CN		
Vestibular		
• Nystagmus	Absent	Absent

- Caloric test—optional
- Postural test—optional

Cochlear

• Finger friction test	N	N
• Tuning fork test (done if any hearing defect is detected by history or finger snapping)		
– Rinne's test	+ve	+ve
– Weber's test	Equal on both sides	
– Schwabach's test	N	N
7. IXth and Xth CN		
• Taste of posterior 2/3 of tongue	Not done	
• Position of uvula and median raphe	Central	
• Movements of palate (say Ah)	Equal	
• Gag reflex	N	N
8. XIth CN		
• Power of sternocleidomastoid	N	N
• Trapezius (shrugging)	N	N
9. XIIth CN		
• Position of tongue on protruding	Central	
• Wasting	Absent	
• Fasciculation (test with tongue inside the mouth)	Absent	
• Power of tongue (test the tongue over the cheek against resistance)	N	N

Motor System

A. Bulk, B. Tone, C. Power (Inspect all muscles and compare first)	N	N

A. Bulk

Measure corresponding points on either sides at forearm, arm, thigh, calf. Also look for wasting of small muscles of hand	N	N

B. Tone

Test flexors and extensors at each joint in each limb	N	N

- *Hypotonia*
  - UMN lesion in neuronal shock

- LMN lesion
- Cerebellar lesion

- *Spasticity*
  - Clasp knife in character
  - Affects antigravity muscles (flexors in UL and extensor in LL), e.g. pyramidal lesions.
- *Rigidity*
  - Lead pipe in character
  - Affects both gravity and antigravity muscles, e.g. extrapyramidal lesion.
    i. When tremor superimposed on rigidity—cogwheel rigidity, e.g. Parkinsonism.

C. Power

1. Upper limb

• Fingers		N	N
• Wrist	Flexion	Grade 5	Grade 5
	Extension	Grade 5	Grade 5
• Elbow	Flexion	Grade 5	Grade 5
	Extension	Grade 5	Grade 5
• Shoulder	Abduction	Grade 5	Grade 5
	Adduction	Grade 5	Grade 5

Trunk

• Beevor's sign		Umbilicus central

2. Lower limb

• Hip	Flexion	Grade 5	Grade 5
	Extension	Grade 5	Grade 5
• Knee	Flexion	Grade 5	Grade 5
	Extension	Grade 5	Grade 5
• Ankle	Dorsiflexion	Grade 5	Grade 5
	Plantar flexion	Grade 5	Grade 5
• Toes	Inversion	N	N
	Eversion	N	N

Power grading—MRC (medical research council)

0 – No movement
1 – Flicker of contraction
2 – Moves with gravity excluded
3 – Moves against gravity, but not against resistance
4 – Moves against gravity and resistance, but not normal
5 – Normal power

Segments	Muscle Groups Paralyzed
C3–C5	Diaphragm
C5	Shoulder abduction
C5–C6	Elbow flexion
C6	Supination, pronation, wrist extension
C7	Wrist flexion, Elbow and finger extension
C8	Finger flexors
T1	Intrinsic hand muscles
T8–T10	Upper abdominal muscles
T10–T12	Lower abdominal muscles
L1–L2	Hip flexors
L2–L3	Hip abduction
L3–L4	Knee extension
L4–L5	Ankle dorsiflexors
L5	Big toe extension
L4, L5, S1	Knee flexion
S1–S2	Ankle and toe flexors
S2–S4	Anal sphincter
S5	Anal reflex

Co-ordination	N	N
Involuntary movements	Absent	
Gait	Normal	

Sensory System

• Superficial sensations		
– Pain	N	N
– Touch	N	N
– Temperature	N	N
• Deep sensations		
– Vibration (128 Hz)		
– Joint position sense	N	N
• *Cortical sensation:* (Test only if primary modalities of sensation are normal)	N	N
– Tactile localization		
– Two point discrimination		
– Stereognosis		
– Graphesthesia		
– Sensory inattention		

Reflexes

• Superficial Reflexes		
– Corneal (CN V and VIII)	N	N
– Abdominal (T7–T12)	N	N
– Cremasteric (L1–L2)	N	N
– Plantar (L5–S1)	Flexor	Flexor
– Anal (S3–S4)	N	N
– Bulbocavernous (S3–54)	N	N
• Deep Tendon Reflexes		
– Jaw jerk	N	N
– Biceps (C5, C6)	N	N
– Supinator (C5, C6)	N	N
– Triceps (C6, C7)	N	N
– Knee jerk (L2, 3, 4)	N	N
– Ankle jerk (S1, S2)	N	N
• Clonus	*Right*	*Left*
– Patellar clonus	Absent	Absent
– Ankle clonus	Absent	Absent

Reflex grading

0 – No movement
1 – Present (N ankle jerk)
2 – Brisk (N knee jerk)
3 – Very brisk
4 – Clonus

Signs of Cerebellar Dysfunction

- Nystagmus
- Staccato (scanning) speech
- Titubation
- Truncal ataxia
- Finger nose test
- Adiadochokinesia
- Heel knee test
- Intention tremor
- Dysmetria
- Tandem walking
- Rebound phenomenon

- Hypotonia
- Pendular knee jerk
- Broad based gait (drunken, reeling)
- *Romberg's sign:* A test of sensory ataxia (not cerebellar ataxia)
- Past pointing
- Dysarthria.

Sign of Meningeal Irritation

- Neck stiffness
- Kernig's sign
- Brudzinsky's
  - Neck sign
  - Leg sign.

Autonomic Nervous System

- Pupil
- Sweating
- Cardiovascular reflex
  - Tachycardia at rest
  - Pulse in Valsalva maneuver and standing
  - BP in standing, hand gripping, stressful tasks
- Postural hypotension—fall of BP by more than 20 mm on standing
- Bladder, bowel
- Impotence.

Skull and Spine

- Swelling
- Tenderness
- Deformity (gibbus)
- Carotid bruit (never forget to look for bruit here and if possible look for ophthalmic bruit also).

Peripheral Nervous System

Look for peripheral nerve thickening.

Trophic Changes

- Trophic ulcers, Charcot's joint, etc.

Blood supply of internal capsule

Recurrent branch: Of ACA
Striate branch: Of MCA
Anterior choroidal artery
Branch: From internal carotid and posterior communicating artery.

Rule of 17

CN V and XII angle of mouth deviated to the paralyzed side 5 + 12
CN VII and X angle of mouth deviated to normal side 7 + 10

Cortical lesion: Seizures
- Aphasia
- Cortical sensory loss
- Primitive reflexes
- Weakness less dense, e.g. faciobrachial monoplegia.

Internal capsule: Contralateral dense hemiplegia
- Contralateral UMN facial palsy
- With or without contralateral hemisensory loss
- Inferior quadrantanopia.

Brainstem: Crossed hemiplegia (i.e. ipsilateral CN with contralateral hemiplegia).

CRANIAL NERVES

- *Motor:* 3, 4, 6, 11, 12
- *Sensory:* 1, 2, 8
- *Others:* Mixed
  - Parasympathetic fibers present in: 3, 7, 9, 10 CNs
  - Midline nuclei CNs—3, 4, 6, 12 (these may be associated with contralateral hemiplegia as corticospinal tract is medial)
  - 4 nuclei of 5th CN
    - Motor—pons
    - Chief sensory—pons (touch, pressure)
    - Mesencephalic nucleus—midbrain (proprioception)
    - Spinal nucleus—C2 to pons (pain and temp)

- 4 nuclei of 7th CN
    - Motor pons
    - Nucleus tractus solitarius—medulla (taste of anterior 1/3 rd of tongue)
    - Superior salivatory—parasympathetic
    - Lacrimatory—parasympathetic.

Examination Tips

The Olfactory Nerve

- Select proper materials: asafetida, coffee powder
- Patient closes his eyes
- Close the opposite nostril
- Ask the patient to take two good sniffs on presenting the substance to the nostril
- Patient tells if he can smell anything
- Ask the patient to identify the substance
- Test the other nostril in the same way.
  [**Comment on:** As normal or abnormal; if abnormal local nasal disease or neural disease, unilateral or bilateral].

The Optic Nerve

- Field of vision (by confrontation)
  - Ask the patient to sit comfortably
  - Sit one meter away facing the patient
  - Ask the patient to close the right eye with his palm and focus the left eye on the tip of your nose
  - Close your left eye and focus right eye on patient's left eye (looking for movements of eyeball)
  - Keep your index finger in mid-position half a meter from the patient's eye
  - Move the finger from periphery to center of the visual field
  - Keep the finger wiggling throughout until patient perceives it
  - Test all four quadrants (comparing with your field).
- Color vision
  - Test each eye separately
  - Use Ishihara's charts or Holmgren's wool.
- Visual acuity (in the absence of Snellen's and near vision charts)
  - Test each eye separately
  - Compare your acuity of vision for progressively distant letters, numbers or objects with that of the patient
  - This gives a rough idea of the patient's acuity assuming that your vision is normal.

The Oculomotor, Trochlear and Abducent Nerves

- Ask for history of diplopia
- Ask the patient to look straight ahead.

Comment on
- The resting position of the eyeball and on squint, if any
- Ptosis, if present
- The pupillary size, if abnormal.

Examine Eyeball Movements

- Use a clear and a definite point (nib of a pen) and ask the patient to follow it
- Move it horizontally to the right and to the left
- Upwards and downwards in the midline
- Upwards and downwards when eyes are deviated to one side
- Examine both eyes
  [**Comment on:** (a) Normal or abnormal; (b) Unilateral or bilateral; (c) The cranial nerve affected].

Light Reflex

- Ask the patient to look at a distance
- Flash bright light from one side
- Note pupillary constriction on the same side (direct light reflex)
- Note pupillary constriction on the opposite side (consensual light reflex)
- Examine both sides.

Accommodation Reflex

- Hold up one finger close to the patient's face
- Ask the patient to look at a distant object
- Assess pupillary size
- Ask the patient to quick look at your finger
- Observe pupillary size now. They will normally constrict.

Trigeminal Nerve

- The motor part inspect for
  - Symmetry of the temporal fossae
  - Symmetry of the angles of the jaw

- Ask the patient to clench her/his teeth:
  i. Palpate temporalis
  ii. Palpate the masseter
- Examine both sides
- Place your hand under the jaw and ask the patient to open her/his mouth against resistance or ask the patient to move her/his jaw from side to side (pterygoids).

Sensory Part

- Explain the procedure to the patient
- Use a wisp of cotton for light touch
- Ask patient to close her/his eyes
- Touch near but not on the midline at the following areas:
  - Forehead
  - Upper part of the sides of the nose
  - Malar regions,
  - Upper lip
  - Chin
  - Anterior part of the tongue (avoid skin over the angle of jaw)
  - Compare with the opposite side
  - Test for pain and temperature sense.

The jaw jerk

- Ask the patient to slightly open her/his mouth
- Place your left forefinger below the patient's lower lip
- Using a knee hammer, gently tap in a downward direction
  Response is an upward jerk of the jaw.

The corneal reflex

- Use a wisp of cotton (moistened with water)
- The patient looks to one side
- Approach the patient's eye from the other side
- Touch at its junction with the sclera
- Examine both sides
- Look for blinking on the same side and on the opposite side.

FACIAL NERVE

Inspection

- Concentrate on symmetry of the face.

- Observe:
  - Face as a whole
  - The wrinkles of the forehead and nasolabial folds
  - The palpebral fissures
  - Movements during talking, smiling, eating and drinking.

Maneuvers

- Ask the patient to wrinkle her/his forehead by looking upwards
- Ask the patient to close both his/her eyes tightly. He resists attempts to open it
- When the patient closes his/her eyes tightly. Look if the eyeballs are seen to turn upwards (Bell's phenomenon)
- Ask the patient to whistle or say 'ooooh'
- Ask the patient to show the teeth or say 'eeee'
- Ask the patient to inflate mouth with air. Tap over each cheek, in turn to check strength
- Ask the patient to evert the lower lip and says 'eeeee' (for platysma).

Taste

- Explain the procedure to the patient
- Use strong solutions of sugar and salt; weak solutions of vinegar or citric acid (sour)
- Ask the patient to protrude out tongue
- Gently hold the tip of the tongue using a gauze
- Moisten the sides of the tongue using solutions with a wooden rod
- The patient indicates the taste by pointing at a card (on which the four possible tastes are written)
- Ask the patient to keep mum during examination
- Ask the patient to cleanse mouth with water after the test
- Repeat the test with another substance
- Examine both sides and compare.

The Auditory Part of VIII Nerve

- Examine the external auditory meatus for wax
- Test one ear at a time, the other ear is tightly closed
- Test with a ticking watch (normally heard within 2 feet)
- Test audibility of a whisper (normally heard within 3 feet).

Rinne's test

- Use a tuning fork of 256 or 512 Hz
- Strike the fork and hold its stem

- Place the base of the fork on the mastoid process and ask the patient if he can hear it vibrating
- Patient tells this when he hears the sound
- Then place the blades near the external auditory meatus
- Patient tells whether he can hear it now or not

  [**Comment on:** Rinne's positive or negative]
  - Rinne's test positive means that air conduction is better than bone conduction.
  - Rinne's negative means that bone conduction is better than air conduction.

Weber's test

- Place the vibrating fork in the midline over the skull or over the mandible.
- Ask the patient whether he can hear the sound equally in both the ears or not

  [Comment as lateralized or to one side]
  - In Weber's test, if the hearing is normal, the sound appears to arise in the midline.
  - If there is nerve deafness, the sound will be lateralized to the healthy side.
  - If there is conduction deafness, the sound is lateralized.

Absolute bone conduction test (ABC test)

- Place the vibrating fork on the patient's mastoid process
- Patient tells when the sound ceases
- Now, place the fork on your mastoid process to compare if you can still hear the sound.

The Vestibular Part of VIII Nerve

- The Caloric test (cold and warm water test)
- Nystagmus.

The Glossopharyngeal and the Vagus Nerve

Elicit history of nasal regurgitation, hoarseness of voice, difficulty in swallowing and choking episodes during eating or drinking.

Motor part

- Ask the patient to say 'egg' or 'rub'
- When the patient opens mouth, tongue is kept on the floor of the mouth. Patient faces the light

- Use a tongue depressor if necessary
- Look for pooling of saliva in the throat
- Note symmetry of the palatal arches and the pharynx
- Ask the patient to say 'ah'
- Observe the movement of palatal arches and the pharynx.

Sensory part (Palatal and pharyngeal reflex)
- Ask the patient to face the light
- Patient opens mouth and keeps the tongue on the floor of the mouth
- Use a tongue depressor, if necessary
- Using a swab, touch the palate or the pharynx on one side
- Note the gag reflex (contraction of palate, pharynx and posterior one-third of the tongue)
- Examine both sides.

The Accessory Nerve

Trapezius

- Ask the patient to elevate the shoulder against resistance (upper one-third)
- Ask the patient to brace and retract the scapula against resistance.
- Palpate the suprascapular region for muscle contraction (middle one-third)
- Ask the patient to push the palms of the hands hard against the wall with elbow fully extended
- Fibers are seen and felt inferior to the angle of the scapulae (lower one-third)
- Accessory nerve supplies only upper one-third of the trapezius. The remaining part is supplied by the C3-C4 segments of the spinal cord
- Examine both sides.

The Hypoglossal Nerve

- Observe when the tongue is resting in the mouth for fasciculation
- Ask the patient to protrude the tongue as far as possible
- Test lateral movement of the tongue by asking the patient to lick all the teeth
- Assess power of the tongue while the patient pushes it against his cheeks
- Palpate the tongue for tone using a gauze piece.

The Motor System

- Bulk of the muscles
  - Compare the bulk of the muscles of both sides by inspection
  - Measure the circumference of the limbs at clearly stated points
  - Examine both sides.
- Tone of the muscles
  - Relax the muscles
  - Palpate the muscle transversely
  - Flex and extend the joint repeatedly
  - Do on both sides and compare.

Clonus

- *Knee clonus:* With the patient relaxed and the knee extended and the skin over knee stretched, sharply push with your thumb and forefinger above the patella towards the foot, sustaining the pressure for few seconds.
- *Ankle clonus:* Support the patient's leg with both the knee and ankle resting in 90 degree flexion. Briskly dorsiflex and partially evert the foot and sustain the pressure.

Strength of the Muscles

- Expose the muscle being tested
- Inspect and palpate the muscle being tested to know that the muscle is contracting
- Position the limb properly. If the adductors of the hip are to be tested, keep the legs fully abducted at the hip at the beginning of the examination so that the full range of adduction can be appreciated
- Examine both sides
- Grade the muscle power.

Superficial Reflexes

- Superficial abdominal reflex
  - Patient lies supine
  - Expose the patient's abdomen
  - Patient keeps his abdominal muscles relaxed
  - Use an atraumatic object, key, wood sticks, knee hammer
  - Lightly stroke the abdomen from the lateral end towards the midline
  - Test all four quadrants Root value (T6–T12).

- Plantar reflex
  - Patient lies supine with legs relaxed
  - Expose the legs adequately till the hip
  - Explain the procedure to the patient
  - Use a blunt object (Tip of knee hammer)
  - Steady the ankle with the other hand
  - Apply firm pressure while stroking
  - Start stroking the sole from the lateral end of the heel
  - Stop short of the ball of the great toe
  - Examine both sides
  - *Root value:* L5, S1.
- Alternate methods
  - *Oppenheim's sign:* Squeezing the calf or pressing heavily along the inner border of the tibia
  - *Gordon's sign:* Pinch the tendo-Achilles
  - *Schaeffer's sign:* Pinch the calf muscles
  - *Bing's sign:* Pricking the dorsum of the foot or great toe with a pin
  - *Gonda's sign:* Do forceful snapping of the second to the fourth toes
  - *Chaddock's sign:* Pinch skin over the lateral malleolus.

Superficial Spinal Reflexes

Reflex	How excited	Clinical result
Anal (S3, S4)	Stroking or scratching skin near anus	Contraction of anal sphincter
Bulbocavernosus (S3, S4)	Pinching dorsum of glans penis	Contraction of bulbo-cavernosus
Plantar response (L5, S1)	Stroking the sole of the foot and toes or leg	Flexion of toes and or foot
Cremasteric (L1, L2)	Stroking the skin at the upper and inner part of thigh	Upward movement of testicle
Abdominal (T7–T12)	Stroking the abdominal wall below coastal margin and in iliac fossa	Contraction of abdominal muscles
Scapular (C5–T1)	Stroking the skin in interscapular region	Contraction of scapular muscles

Deep Reflexes

Biceps jerk

- Ask the patient to lie supine or sit up
- Patient's elbow is flexed to about 90 degree and is supported
- The forearm is semipronated
- Place your thumb or index finger on the biceps tendon
- Using the knee hammer strike on your own finger
- *Root value:* C5, C6.

Triceps jerk

- Patient lies supine
- Patient's forearm is drawn across the trunk and is allowed to lie over his abdomen
- The arm is well-exposed
- Strike directly 2–5 cm above the elbow
- *Root value:* C6, C7.

Supinator jerk

- Patient lies supine or sits up
- The elbow is flexed and supported
- The forearm is exposed and placed in the semiproned position
- Strike over the distal end of the radius about 4 cm above the wrist joint (on the styloid process)
- *Root value:* C5, C6.

  [**Comment on:** Jerk is said to be inverted when there is absent contraction of the biceps and brachioradialis but finger flexion occurs].

Knee jerk

- Patient lies supine
- Quadriceps is exposed
- Knees supported and flexed to about 15–30 degree
- Sharply tap the patellar tendon
- *Root value:* L2, L3, L4.

Ankle jerk

- Ask the patient to lie supine
- Expose the calf muscles
- Lower limb is abducted and externally rotated at the hip and slightly flexed at the knee
- Slightly dorsiflex the foot and the ankle
- Strike the posterior aspect of the Achilles tendon
- *Root value:* S1, S2.

Released Reflexes/Primitive Reflexes

- Palmomental reflex
- Grasp reflex
- Glabellar tap reflex
- Snout reflex
- Sucking reflex.

Cerebellar Function Tests

Finger nose test

- Patient holds the hand outstretched and abducted to 90 degree at the shoulder
- Patient touches the tip of the nose with the help of his index finger
- The finger is held on to the nose (to a count of five)
- Repeat the test 2 or 3 times on both the sides.

Dysdiadochokinesia

- Patient does rapid alternating movements—with the elbow flexed the forearm supinated and pronated
- The patient slaps the palm with the front and back of the other hand.

Heel knee test

- Patient's heel is placed on the opposite knee
- The heel is slide accurately down the front of the shin to the ankle and back again
- Repeat the test with the other heel.

Walking along the straight line

- Patient walks along the straight line
- He/she places the heel of one foot immediately in front of the great toe of the one behind
- He/she goes forward and turns to come back.

Romberg's sign

- Patient stands with his/her feet close together
- Tries to stay still with the eyes closed.

Sensory System

Pain

- Superficial pain
  - Use the point of a pin as a stimulus
  - Look at the patient's face while testing with pricks.

- Deep pain
  - Squeeze the muscle or tendon
  - Look at the patient's face for the response.

Temperature

- Use ideal warm temperature (37–40) and ideal cold temperature (30–32) as far as possible
- Use 2 identical test tubes
- Use the test tubes in sequence.

Fine touch

- Use a wisp of cotton or the tip of your index finger
- Touch the skin lightly.

Joint position sense

- Ask the patient to close the eyes
- Hold the joint by the sides
- Move the digit by about 15–30 degree only (avoid alternate movements)
- Give credibility to persistent correct response
- Examine the fingers and toes.

Vibration sense

- Use a 128 Hz tuning fork
- Ask the patient to close the eyes
- Fork is placed on bony prominences
- Start with distal bony prominences
- Examine more proximal areas next.

Cortical Sensations

Graphesthesia

- Use a blunt object (so as not to cause pain)
- Draw legible numbers on the patient's skin
- Try easy numbers first—1, 7, 2
- Try tougher ones next—0, 6, 8.

Steriognosis

- Ask the patient to close both the eyes
- Place a familiar object on the patient's palms like coins, keys, pen, wallet
- Wait for the patient to recognize the object only by touch
- Compare the speed and accuracy of response on both sides.

Two-point discrimination

- Use 2 similar blunt object
- Start by keeping them far apart on the skin
- Bring them closer until patient recognizes them as one
- Examine fingers, palm, foot and back
- Examine both sides and compare identical areas.

Touch localization

- Touch some points on the patient's body with a blunt object
- Patient should show the point touched with his forefinger.

Signs of Meningeal Irritation

Neck stiffness

- Patient actively flexes his neck as fully as he can and then relaxes
- Then passively flex the neck (normally the chin should touch the chest without causing pain).

Kernig's sign

- The patient is made to lie supine
- The opposite leg is fully extended
- Flex the hip to 90 degrees on the same side
- Passively extend the patient's knee.

Brudzkinski's sign

- Flex the head
- The thighs and knees also flex
- Flex one thigh fully
- The opposite thigh also flexes.

Examination of an Unconscious Patient

History

- Enquire whether the bystander was present at the time the patient lost consciousness?
- Find out what exactly was he doing at the time of onset or just before?
- Was the incident abrupt or not?
- Ask whether he had?
  - Headache, vomiting, convulsion before he became unconscious
  - Taken any drugs/poison
  - Whether diabetic, hypertensive or suffering from cardiac or renal diseases
  - Whether he had repeated vomiting or diarrhea before the attack (electrolyte intolerance)

- Whether he had recurrent history of TIA
- Whether alcoholic-hepatic encephalopathy
- Whether any thyroid disease—myxedema, coma.

General Examination

Whether any wound or any injury to the head/discharge from the ear?

Attitude of the patient

- Decorticate
- Decerebrate
- Unilateral movement of limbs/paucity of movement on any side
- Involuntary movement
- Pallor—CRF
- Jaundice—hepatic encephalopathy
- Cyanosis—cardiac lesion
- Thyroid swelling and signs of hypothyroidism with nonpitting edema
- Pedal edema (pitting)—CRF, CCF, liver diseases.

Vital Signs

- Respiratory rate—Any pattern like Cheyne-Stokes respiration
- *BP:* High BP
- *Pulse:* Any arrhythmia, bradycardia
- *Temperature:* Pyrexia-pontine hemorrhage

Try to grade the patient according to Glasgow coma scaling of the person (EMV).

Higher functions: Give importance to speech.

Cranial Nerves

I. - Not checked

II. - If opening the eye, look for menace reflex which helps in roughly assessing the visual acuity, visual field, and VIIth nerve.

III, IV, VI. - Look for doll's eye movement which helps in assessing the range of movement also.

- *It has 2 inferences:*
  1. The inhibition by cortex is lost (normally inhibited by cortex).
  2. Brainstem is intact.
     Very important—pupils size, shape, symmetry, light reflex (no accommodation reflex)

VII. 1. - Menace reflex

2. - Apply pain stimulation (*) and look for deviation of mouth and closure of lips
[*- Pain stimulation can be applied by pressing at the root of orbit or rubbing over the sternum (without the bystanders knowing what you are doing)]

VIII. - Startle reflex (clapping loudly near the ear)

IX., X. - Look for nasogastric tube (indicating aspiration or inability to swallow)

- If mouth is open, we can do gag reflex (but it is dangerous)

XI. - Look for head movement and try to resist it

XII. - Look for wasting and fasciculation if the mouth is open.

Motor: Power: See if the patient is raising his limb against gravity and try to resist it. Rest is same.

Sensory: Only pain sensation can be tested.

Cerebellar signs cannot be tested: As power is less than grade 3 and also the commands cannot be obeyed.

Signs of Meningeal Irritation

- Remember that if the signs are unilateral, it is most probable of organic origin while if bilateral, it may be metabolic in origin (except hypoglycemia which may present in any form)
- Tics and jerks are common if cause is metabolic
- While investigating these patients; always look for blood glucose and electrolyte levels.

Glasgow Coma Scale

Eyes open	Spontaneously	4
	To verbal command	3
	To painful stimulus	2
	Do not open	1
Verbal	Normal, oriented, conversation	5
	Confused	4
	Inappropriate/words only	3
	Sounds only	2

Contd...

Contd...

	No sounds	1
	Intubated patient	T
Motor	Obeys commands	6
	Localizes to pain	5
	Withdrawal/flexion	4
	Abnormal flexion (decorticate)	3
	Extension (decerebrate)	2
	No motor response	1

Causes of Coma with Neck Stiffness

- Subarachnoid hemorrhage
- Meningitis—bacterial and viral (aseptic)
- Encephalitis
- Intracerebral hemorrhage
- Cerebral malaria.

Causes of Coma with Hyperventilation

- Metabolic acidosis
- Diabetic ketoacidosis
- Brainstem lesion, e.g. stroke
- Rising intracranial pressure
- Bacterial meningitis
- Renal failure
- Liver failure
- Pneumonia complicating brain lesion.

Causes of Coma with Focal Neurological Signs

- Epilepsy (postictal stage)
- Stroke
- Encephalitis
- Subarachnoid hemorrhage
- Cerebral abscess
- Bacterial meningitis with cortical infarction
- Cerebral venous sinus thrombosis.

Persistent Vegetative State

- No evidence of awareness of self or environment
- All responses are reflex in nature
- No meaningful or voluntary response to stimulation
- No evidence of language comprehension or expression
- An intermittent sleep/wake pattern
- Preserved cranial nerve responses
- Sufficiently intact hypothalamic (brainstem) autonomic function to allow prolonged survival with nursing and medical care
- Present for more than one month.

2 Surgery Format

SWELLING OR LUMP

History of Present Illness

- *Duration:* Shorter-benign
- *Longer:* Malignant
- *Mode of onset:* Sudden or gradual
- Associated symptoms
- *Pain:* Nature, site, time of onset, radiation, difficulty in respiration/ swallowing
- Fever
- Impairment of function
- *Progress of swelling:* Stationary or continued
- History of trauma
- *Secondary changes:* Softening, ulceration, fungation, inflammatory changes
- *History of recurrence:* Malignant—recurs after removal
- *Cystic swelling:* If cyst wall not completely removed
- History of loss of appetite and weight loss.

History of Past Illness

Similar illness: TB, syphilis. History of surgery.

Personal History

- Betel chewing (nut, slaked lime, tobacco) responsible for growth in cheek, tongue, mouth, lip.
- History of alcohol intake.

Family History

Similar illness: TB, von Recklinghausen's disease, malignancy

General Examination

PICCLE (Pallor, icterus, cyanosis, clubbing, lymph node enlargement, edema).

Vitals
L/E **(Local examination)**.

Inspection

- Site
- Shape
- Size
- *Surface:* Cauliflower (squamous cell carcinoma) irregular numerous branched (papilloma)
- Extent
- *Color:* Blue (ranula); black (nevus, melanoma); red (hemangioma)
- *Margin:* Well defined, poorly defined
- Number
- Pulsation
- *Impulse on cough:* Meningocele, hernia
- *Moving with deglutition:* Thyroid swelling
- Skin over swelling
- Any sinuses, scar, prominent veins.

Palpation

- Local rise of temperature and tenderness
- Site, size, shape, number, extent, surface, margin
- Consistency
- Fluctuation
- Transillumination
- Impulse on cough
- Pulsatility-transmitted (swelling superficial to artery); expansile (originates from arterial wall)
- Reducibility
- Compressibility
- Fixity to overlying skin-papilloma, epithelioma, sebaceous cyst
- Skin over the swelling-pinchable (if not fixed to skin)
- Relation to superficial and deep part-skin, subcutaneous tissue, muscle, tendon, bone, joint, vessels.

Examination of Regional Lymph Node

Site, size, tenderness, number, texture, fixity, matted/not

Percussion

- Shifting dullness
- Fluid thrill
- Percussion note over swelling.

Auscultation

- Bowel sounds, succussion splash-abdominal swelling
- Bruit-aneurysm.

Measurements

Compare with opposite side in case of wasting

Movements

Examine the movement of nearby joints.

Examination of Pressure Effects

- Arterial pulse-weak distal to swelling
- Nerve-wasting, paresis, paralysis
- Vein-distal edema, venous engorgement.

Diagnosis

- Anatomical location
- Pathological nature
- Complication.

Anatomical Pathological

Skin, subcutaneous tissue, muscle, tendon, bones, joints, congenital, traumatic, inflammatory—acute and chronic, vessels, arteries, neoplasm—benign and malignant.

Example

Lipoma—this person is having benign subcutaneous tissue swelling probably lipoma without any features of complication.

3 Ortho Format

HISTORY OF PRESENT ILLNESS

Age

- Green-stick fracture in children
- Dislocation is common in adults.

Amount and nature of violence—

- If the violence is not severe enough to cause fracture then it is a pathological fracture.
- Nature of violence is of three types—Direct, indirect and muscular.
  - Direct—Tapping and crushing
  - Indirect—Twisting, bending, bending force with axial compression
  - Muscular—Patella, olecranon, lesser trochanter of femur.

Pain

- Fracture causes less pain than a sprain or strain
- In dislocation pain is constant and unbearable till it is reduced
  - Loss of function
  - Deformity or swelling.

HISTORY OF PAST ILLNESS

History of tuberculosis, trauma, bacillary dysentery, bleeding diathesis, enteric fever, sore throat, sexual exposure (STD induced arthritis or reactive arthritis), urethritis.

Family History

History of tuberculosis, hemophilia or gout.

OCCUPATIONAL HISTORY

Local Examination

Inspection

- Abnormal swelling and deformity
- Attitude
- Shortening
- Overlying skin—whether exposed as in compound or open fracture.

Palpation

- Tenderness—Bony tenderness due to fracture is called local bony tenderness
- In joint injuries the maximum point of tenderness is noted to know the structures involved
- Bony irregularity—Definite sign of fracture
- Abnormal movements—Definite sign of fracture
- Crepitus
- Pain elicited by manipulating from a distance—Rotating; squeezing or giving axial pressure
- Absence of transmitted movements
- Swelling and wound.

Measurement

- Longitudinal
- Measurement of circumference of limb.

Movements

- Active and passive movements are tested of nearby joints
- Restricted movements or excessive mobility
- Any pain on movement
- Crepitus or grating sensation on movement
- Any associated muscular spasm.

Reflexes

Root values of tendon reflexes

Root value	Tendon reflex
C5	Biceps
C6	Brachioradialis
C7	Triceps
L3, 4	Quadriceps
L5, S1	Achilles tendon

General Examination

Look for Vitals

Minimal screen for locomotor system—(GALS)

- *Gait:* Look for symmetry, walking aids, stiffness, transfers, speed
- *Arms:* Inspection of all surfaces (soft tissue swelling, effusion, muscle wasting), power grip, pinch grip, flexion/extension of elbows, place hands behind head with elbows right back
- *Legs:* Inspection (as above), callosities on feet, flexion/extension of the knees and rotation of the hips
- *Spine:* Rotation, flexion, extension and lateral flexion of neck and lumbar spine looking for any evidence of discomfort as well as restricted movement. Palpation and percussion for local tenderness.

General examination of the spine

Inspection and palpation—Look for tenderness, mobility, kyphoscoliosis and gibbus.

Mobility of the spine and individual joints

- Cervical spine
  - *Rotation:* Ask the patient to look over one, then the other shoulder
  - *Flexion:* Ask the patient to touch chin to the chest
  - *Extension:* Ask the patient to look up to the ceiling
  - *Lateral bending:* Ask the patient to bend the neck sideways and to try to touch the shoulder with the ear without raising the shoulder.
- Thoracic and lumbar spine
  - *Flexion:* Ask the patient to try to touch their toes without bending at the knees
  - *Extension:* Ask the patient to bend backwards

  - *Lateral bending:* Ask the patient to run the hand down the side of the thigh as far as possible
  - *Thoracic rotation:* Ask the seated patient, with arms crossed, to twist round to the left and right as far as possible.
- *Sacroiliac joints:* Tests for irritability
  - Direct pressure over each sacroiliac joint
  - Firm pressure with the side of the hand over the sacrum
  - Inward pressure over both iliac bones in an attempt to distort the pelvis
  - Flex the hip to 90 degrees and exert firm pressure at the knees through the femoral shaft (this should only be done if the knee is not painful).
- Shoulder
  - Flexion
  - Extension
  - Abduction
  - Rotation in abduction
  - Rotation in neutral position
  - Elevation (also involving scapular movement).
- Elbow
  - Flexion
  - Hyperextension.
- Forearm
  - Supination
  - Pronation.
- Wrist
  - Dorsiflexion (extension)
  - Palmar flexion
  - Ulnar deviation
  - Radial deviation.
- Fingers
  - Flexion at MCP, PIP and DIP joints.
- Thumb
  - Extension
  - Flexion (measured as for fingers)
  - Opposition
  - Abduction (movement at right angles to the plane of palm).
- Hand
  - Deformities in joint disease—swan neck and boutonniere deformity

- Deformities due to neuropathy—wasting of thenar and hypothenar eminence and loss of sensations of palmar and dorsal aspects of hand
- Assessment of hand function—test hand grip and pinch grip (between index and thumb).

- Hip
  - *Flexion:* Measured with knee bent. Opposite thigh must remain in neutral position. Flex the knee as the hip flexes
  - *Abduction:* Measured from a line which forms an angle of 90 degrees with a line joining the anterior superior iliac spines
  - Adduction (measured in the same manner)
  - Rotation in flexion
  - Rotation in extension
  - *Extension:* Attempt to extend the hip with the patient lying in the lateral position
  - *Additional examination:* Test for flexion deformity (Thomas test); Trendelenburg test and measurement of true and apparent shortening.
- Knee
  - *Inspection:* (complete extension is the neutral position). Observe for valgus or varus deformities; muscle wasting; joint swelling
  - *Test for stability:* Anterior drawer test, posterior drawer test, etc.
- Ankle
  - *Dorsiflexion:* Test with the knee in flexion and extension to exclude tight calf muscles
  - *Plantar flexion:* Place a finger on the head of the talus to be sure that it is moving. A hypermobile subtalar joint can mimic movement in an arthrodesed ankle.
- Foot
  - *Subtalar inversion and eversion:* Cup the heel in the hands and move it in relation to the tibia without any up and down movement; this eliminates movements at the ankle or midtarsal joints
  - *Midtarsal inversion/eversion and adduction/abduction:* Hold the os calcis in the neutral position in one hand and grasp the forefoot in the other
  - Metatarsophalangeal and interphalangeal flexion/extension.

Systemic Examination

To search for evidences of pleurisy, pericarditis, vasculitis, hepatosplenomegaly, aortic incompetence or lymphadenopathy.

Investigations

- Routine examination
- Specific examination
  - X-ray examination—two views are anteroposterior and lateral
  - Serum Ca
  - Alkaline phosphatase
  - Acid phosphatase
  - Urine-Bence Jones protein in multiple myeloma
  - Bone scan
  - Arthroscopy
  - Arthrography.

Diagnosis

- *Fracture:* Diagnosed by history of trauma; localized pain; swelling and deformity; local bony tenderness; local bony irregularity; crepitus and X-ray.
- *Dislocation:* Diagnosed by deformity; abnormal swelling near a joint; rigidity of joints in passive movements and X-ray.
- *Sprain:* Diagnosed by presence of tenderness on the ligament particularly at the bony attachment; passive stretching of the ligament causes excruciating pain; no local bony tenderness or local bony irregularity; X-ray shows no bony injury.

Points noted in X-ray

- Situation, line of fracture, displacement
- Signs of union in old fracture
- Sclerosis in the fracture end with a gap in between nonunion
- Myositis ossificans and avascular necrosis.

Discussion

Pathological fracture: A fracture through a bone which has been made weak by some underlying disease.

Causes of pathological fracture are:

- *In infants:* Osteogenesis imperfecta (dwarfism, broad skull, blue sclera, scoliosis, ligament laxity, otosclerosis); osteopetrosis
- *In children:* Acute osteomyelitis, solitary bone cysts
- *Young adults:* Osteoclastoma, osteosarcoma
- *Adults:* Generalized fibrocystic disease (hyperparathyroidism); multiple myeloma
- *Elderly:* Senile osteoporosis; Paget's disease and secondary carcinoma.

4 Antenatal Case Format

ANTENATAL CASE TAKING FORMAT

Name	
Age	
Address	
Occupation	
Name and occupation of husband	
Income	
Blood group if Rh(–)ve	

Obstetric formula (G, P, L, A)

- Primigravida if first pregnancy (Elderly primi > 30 years) or
- ______ gravida, para ______ with ______ living children ______ abortions.
- With last menstrual period on ______ and expected date of confinement ______ cycles being regular. (It would be preferable to mention the PLMP)
- Last child birth ______ years ago.
- Date of admission.

Presenting complaints

- Admitted for safe confinement (in these cases do not mention presenting complaints)
- Pain/bleeding/leaking/decreased fetal movements
- Found to have high BP/IUGR/high blood sugar/edema/convulsions/hyperemesis.

History of present illness (Omit if for safe confinement):

Onset, progress, duration, associated symptoms (some teachers prefer to go directly to the history of present pregnancy and mention the complaints in detail in the appropriate trimester while others prefer a chronological order like menstrual history followed by marital followed by past obstetric history, followed by present obstetric history. You stick on to the pattern taught in your unit).

History of Present Pregnancy

- 1st trimester (< 12 weeks)
  - Detected to be pregnant ______ weeks after missing her periods by urine pregnancy test.
    Since then she had regular antenatal check-up.
  - Pain
  - Excessive vomiting
  - Bleeding
  - Fever with rash
  - Drugs/radiation
  - Urinary tract infections
  - TT (both doses)
  - Folic acid
- IInd trimester (13–28 weeks)
  - Quickening felt at _____ weeks
  - USG taken at _____ month
  - Hypertension
  - Diabetes
  - UTI
  - Bleeding
  - Over distension
  - Edema
  - Iron folic acid and calcium tablets
- IIIrd trimester (>28 weeks)
  - Bleeding/Leaking/Discharge/decreased fetal movements
  - Pain
  - Edema/hypertension (PIH)
  - Diabetes (GDM)
  - Varicosity.

Past Obstetric History (In Chronological Order of Previous Pregnancies)

Home/hospital; Vaginal/CS (indication): FTND/PTD/IUD/ABN: Vacuum/forceps birth weight; any postnatal complications: Prolonged hospital stay; any neonatal resuscitation required. Condition and age of the babies at present.

Menstrual History

- Menarche (age) LMP, PLMP
- Rhythm (regular or not)

- Length of the cycle
- Duration of flow
- Amount of flow
- Premenstrual symptoms
- Associated pain.

Marital History

- Age at marriage
- Duration of marriage
- Frequency of coitus
- Dyspareunia
- Contraceptive method adopted
- Treatment for infertility.

Past History

- Any chronic illness (DM, thyroid, TB, HTN)
- Any surgical interventions (D and C, D and E)
- Any drug intake.

Family History

- Chronic illnesses and malignancies
- Congenital anomalies/repeated abortions
- Multiple pregnancies.

Personal History

- Any addictions
- Diet
- Bowel and bladder habits
- History of Anti-D Ig in case of Rh (–)ve mothers.

Treatment History

History of allergy to drugs.

General Examination

Height, weight and gait are a must.

- Built and nourishment
- Posture and attitude
- Pallor, jaundice, cyanosis, clubbing

- LNE, pedal edema, varicosities
- Skin, hair and nails
- Thyroid and breast
- **Vital signs:** Pulse, BP, respiration, temperature

Other Systems

- CVS, respiratory system, GIT, CNS
- Obstetric examination (after evacuation of bladder)

Inspection

- Abdomen longitudinally distended
- Flanks are full/empty
- Striae gravidarum and linea nigra seen
- Scars/engorged veins/shiny skin if present
- Umbilicus is central inverted/everted.

Palpation (with legs semiflexed)

- Fundal height (in cm corresponds to gestational age between 18 and 32 weeks)
- Symphisiofundal height
- Abdominal girth (> 100 cm abnormal)

  Leopold's maneuvers
- Fundal grip
  - Hard, round, freely movable and ballotable mass-corresponds to **head**
  - Broad, soft, irregular, nonballotable—corresponds to **breech**
  - In **oblique** lie the pole is shifted to one side
  - In **extended breech** the head is nonballotable due to splintage
  - In **transverse lie** the spine or fetal parts may be obtained.
- Umbilical grip
  - Firm, uniform resistance—**Back**
  - Multiple nodules—**Limbs**
  - If the nodules are felt on both sides, probably the back is posteriorly—placed and limbs anteriorly.
- First pelvic grip
  - To know the presenting part
  - Hard, round—**Cephalic**
  - Soft, broad—**Breech**
  - Empty—**Oblique lie**
  - Head fixed or not

- Second pelvic grip
  - Confirm the findings of the first pelvic grip
  - Whether engaged (only one prominence palpable) or not (both prominences palpable, i.e. occiput and sinciput).
  - If cephalic whether **Flexed** (occiput at a lower level than sinciput) or **Deflexed** (occiput at a higher level)
  - No need of this grip, if first pelvic grip is empty.

Auscultation

FHS heard below/above umbilicus on left/right side
FHR = rate/min

- To ascertain whether fetus alive or not
- To locate the position of fetus
- Breech above umbilicus
- Cephalic-below umbilicus
- Normal fetal heart rate 120–160/min.

SUMMARY

_______ year old GPLA at gestational age of _______ weeks (with LMP on _______ and EDC on _______,) admitted for _______ with history of _______ complications with previous FTND/LSCS _______ years ago; mention any significant history of GDM, PIH, APH, blood transfusion. On examination (o/e) pallor, edema, vital signs and system examination. Obstetric examination-singleton, longitudinal line, cephalic presentation with good FHS.

Diagnosis

Twenty-two years old primigravida at 37 weeks of gestation (with expected date of confinement on...). On examination vertex presentation, head not engaged. Fetal heart sound heard. Complications if any.

Fundal height	Weeks
Just above symphysis	12
Midway between umbilicus and symphysis	16
Umbilicus lower border	20

Contd ...

Contd ...

Just above umbilicus	24
Lower 3rd between xiphi-umbilicus	28
Middle 3rd between xiphi-umbilicus	32
At xiphi flanks not full	36
Middle 3rd between xiphi-umbilicus + flank full	40

Johnson's Formula (when vertex at ischial spine)
Fetal weight in g = (Fundal height – 12) × 155 g

Dawns Formula
Uterine volume (mL) = fundal height × 1.36 mL

5 Gynecology Case Format

GYNECOLOGY CASE TAKING FORMAT

Name	
Age	
Address	
Occupation	
Income	

PRESENTING COMPLAINTS

- Discharge PV
  - Amount (Profuse/scanty)
  - Color (whitish/greenish/blood stained)
  - Nature (mucoid/curdy/frothy)
  - Odor (offensive/urinary)
  - Relation to menstrual cycle
  - Associated symptoms (burning pain)
  - Association with micturition/defecation
- Bleeding PV
  - Amount and number of days (Number of pads she had to use)
  - Relation to menstruation
  - Passage of clots
  - Associated pain/discharge/fever
- Pain
  - Relation with menstrual cycle
  - Nature, intensity, onset, location
  - Relation to food, posture, urination
  - Aggravating and relieving factors
  - Other associations
  - Fever

Causes of discharge

• *Cervicitis:* Milky white viscoid • *Candida:* White curdy • Trichomoniasis frothy yellowish green • Pyogenic foul smelling brownish • Neoplasms blood stained • Foreign body foul smelling watery • Fistula urinary and fecal
Oligomenorrhea Infrequent menstruation occurring at intervals >35 days
Hypomenorrhea Decrease amount of flow (normal 50–80 mL)
Polymenorrhea (Epimenorrhea) Frequent cycles of intervals < 21 days
Metrorrhagia Irregular intermenstrual vaginal bleeding in between apparently normal periods

- Dyspareunia
  - Superficial/deep
  - Primary/secondary
- Infertility
  - Primary/secondary
  - Frequency and timing of coitus
- Urinary symptoms
  - Burning pain
  - Frequency
  - Retention
  - Incontinence
  - Enuresis
- Bowel symptoms
  - Constipation
  - Diarrhea

  Menstrual history
  - Menarche (age) LMP, PLMP
  - Rhythm (regular or not)
  - Length of the cycle
  - Duration of flow
  - Amount of flow
  - Premenstrual symptoms
  - Associated pain
  - Menopausal symptoms/menopause

Marital history
- Age at marriage
- Duration of marriage
- Frequency of coitus
- Dyspareunia
- Contraceptive method adopted
- Treatment for infertility

Obstetric history
- No of deliveries
- Type of delivery (Normal/cesarian/home/hospital)
- Birthweight of babies
- Any abortions (If yes, duration/spontaneous/method)
- Last child birth.

1° dysmenorrhea (Spasmodic/intrinsic)

Severe intermittent colicky pain on the first day (Few hours or a day before the onset of bleeding) rarely lasting for > 12 hours.

2° dysmenorrhea (Congestive/extrinsic)

Begins up to 5 days premenstrually. Dull pain in the lower back or abdomen and relieved with the onset of menstruation.

Past History

- Any chronic illness (DM, thyroid, TB, HTN)
- Any surgical interventions (D and C, D and E)
- Any drug intake.

Family History

- Chronic illnesses and malignancies
- Congenital anomalies/repeated abortions
- Multiple pregnancies.

Personal History

- Any addictions
- Diet
- Bowel and bladder habits.

General Examination

- Built and nourishment (Height and weight)
- Posture and attitude

- Pallor, jaundice, cyanosis, clubbing
- LNE, pedal edema, varicosities
- Skin, hair and nails
- Thyroid and breast
- *Vital signs:* Pulse, BP, respiration, temperature.

Other Systems

- CVS
- Respiratory system
- Nervous system
- Gastrointestinal system.

Abdominal Examination (After Evacuation of the Bladder)

Inspection

- Shape, distension and movement with respiration
- Umbilicus, pulsations, veins, scars, striae
- Visible swelling—shape, size, site, edges, pressure effects.

Palpation

- Temperature, tenderness, guarding, rigidity.
- Swelling-number, size, site, shape, surface, skin over the swelling, borders, mobility, consistency
  - Liver
  - Spleen
  - Lumbar spine.

Percussion

- Note over swelling
- Liver span
- Traube's space.

Auscultation

- Bruit
- Bowel sounds.

Summary

Diagnosis

6 Pediatrics Case Format

CLINICAL CASE TAKING FORMAT

Name	
Age	
DoB	
Sex	
Address	
Informant (Reliable or not)	

Presenting Complaints

Mention in chronological order

- History of present illness (*Note:* Never use the term history of presenting complaints)
- *Onset:* Sudden, gradual, insidious
- *Progress:* Increasing, decreasing
- Relapsing/recurring
- Character of each symptom—aggravating and relieving factors
- Associated symptoms
- Enquire about the rest of the cardinal symptoms and mention (Even if absent).

History of Past Illness

- History of similar illness in the past (If yes describe in detail)
- History of any vaccine preventable diseases especially mumps, measles and TB
- Any other cause of morbidity in the past like recurrent respiratory tract infections/diarrhea.

Antenatal History

Refer obstetrics case format.

Natal History

- *Type of delivery:* Term/preterm
- Normal instrumental cesarian (Indication)
- Presentation
- Complications, if any
- *Place of delivery:* Home/hospital.

Postnatal History

- First cry
- Birth weight
- Any resuscitation required
- Passage of meconium/urine
- Seizures/jaundice
- Exchange transfusion.

Developmental History

Gross motor development

Neck holding	3 months
Supine to prone	5 months
Sitting without support	8 months
Standing without support	12 months
Walking without support	13 months
Running	18 months
Walking upstairs	24 months

Fine motor development

Grasps rattle	4 months
Reaching out	5 months
Palmar grasp	6 months
Transfer objects	7 months
Pincer grasp	9 months

Linguistic development

Turns head to sound	1 month
Cooing	3 months

Contd ...

Contd ...

Monosyllables (ma, ba)	6 months
Bisyllables (mama, baba)	9 months
2 words with meaning	15 months
10 words with meaning	18 months
Simple story	24 months
Telling a story	36 months

Social and adaptive development

Social smile	2 months
Smile of recognition	3 months
Smiles at mirror	5 months
Stranger anxiety	7 months
Waves bye bye	10 months

Bowel and bladder control

Bowel control	12 months
Bladder control (dry by day)	24 months
(dry by night)	36 months

Fine motor skills

1.5 years	Scribble
2 years	Draw a line
3 years	Draw a circle
4 years	Rectangle or '+' sign
5 years	Triangle or 'x' sign
6 years	Hexagon

At 1 year

- Walk like a bear
- Bottom shuffling
- Walk with one hand support
- Casting
- Turn 2 to 3 pages of a book
- Mimics mother
- Utter 2 words with meaning

At 2 years

- Climbing stairs (2 feet on 1 step)
- Running
- Screwing
- Turns pages one by one
- Draw a line
- Say simple sentences

At 3 years

- Climbing stairs (1 foot at a time)
- Stands on one leg
- Handedness
- Tricycle
- Assemble toys
- Able to dress and undress
- Draw a circle
- 250 words—telling

Red flag sign in child development

Milestone	Age
No visual fixation by	2 months
No vocalization by	6 months
Not sitting without support by	9–10 months
Not standing alone by	16 months
Not walking alone by	18 months
No single words by	18 months
Loss of imaginative play	3 years
Loss of comprehension, single words or phrases	At any age

Hearing and Vision

Mention whether the development of the child is normal in all spheres of development and whether it comparable with his/her siblings. In case of any developmental delay, mention must be made on the developmental age of the child. Mention whether there is any deviation from normal development or regression of any milestones.

Immunization History

- Fully immunized to date or not according to the National Immunization schedule
- Look for BCG scar
- Last vaccine taken
- Booster doses of any vaccine
- Pulse polio status
- Any optional vaccines taken, if so why.

National immunization schedule

At birth	BCG, OPV
6 weeks	DPT, OPV
10 weeks	DPT, OPV
14 weeks	DPT, OPV
9 months	Measles
18 months	OPV, DPT booster
4–5 years	DT booster

Dietetic History

- Whether prelacteal feeds given or not
- When put to breast
- Exclusively breast fed till ________
- Weaning at ________ months with ________
- Breastfeeding stopped at ________
- Started sharing the family diet at ________
- Any dietary modification advised as the part of treatment (Say nephrotic syndrome)
- Calculate daily caloric and protein intake (See the table given later) according to new ICMR recommendation
- Comment whether caloric and protein adequate/inadequate
- Mention about any inadequacy.

(Say iron rich food in anemia or green leaf vegetables in vitamin deficiency).

Family History

- Draw the pedigree chart
- Age of parents (especially in congenital condition's like Down's)

- Consanguinity
- Other chronic illnesses in the family
- Similar illnesses in the family
- Siblings and their diseases
- History of repeated abortions/still births.

Socioeconomic History

- Occupation of parents and income, housing, surroundings
- Education of parents
- Sanitation and environment.

General Examination

General Attitude

- *Physical attitude:* Bedridden/Walking/playful/active/restless/comfortable
- *Mental attitude:* Consciousness/cooperative/nature of cry.

Head to Foot Examination

Pallor, jaundice, cyanosis, clubbing, pedal edema, lymphadenopathy, skin, hair and nails. Other than these, mention any other positive finding you get on examining the patient and specifically look for any stigmatas of vitamin or mineral deficiency; congenital anomalies; any infectious disease; any invasive procedures done (like a Ryles tube or an IV cannula) and so on.

Vital Signs

Pulse, blood pressure, respiration, temperature, jugular venous pressure.

Age	Temp °C	Pulse/min	Resp/min	BP mm Hg
Newborn	36–37	140	40	60/40
Up to 1 year	36.5–17.5	120	30	70/50
Up to 5 years	37+/–0.2	100	20	90/50
Up to 10 years	37+/–0.2	90	18	100/70
>10 years	37+/–0.2	80	18	110/80

Anthropometry

Weight

At birth	2.8–3 kg
At 1 year	9 kg
At 2 years	12 kg
At 3 years	14 kg
1 Standard deviation = 12.5 percent of the value	

Indian academy of pediatrics (IAP) classification of PEM

Above 80 percent of expected normal
71–80% Grade I PEM
61–70% Grade II PEM
51–60% Grade III PEM
<50% Grade IV PEM
(Prefix k if edema is present)

Weight gain

0–3 months	30 g/day
3–6 months	20 g/day
6–9 months	12 g/day
>1 year	250 g/month
>3 years	2 kg/year

Height (Up to 2 years length is taken)

At birth	50 cm
At 1 year	75 cm
At 2 years	87.5 cm
At 3 years	94 cm
At 4 years	100 cm
After 4 years	5–5.5 cm/year
1 Standard deviation = 4 percent of the value	
Short stature <2 Standard deviation	
If patient is too tall or too short then the arm span and upper segment lower segment ratio must be taken.	

Welcome classification

Weight for age	Nutritional status
60–80% no edema	Undernutrition
60–80% with edema	Kwashiorkor
<60% no edema	Marasmus
<60% with edema	Marasmic kwashiorkor

Formula for weight

Age	Weight
3 months–1 year	(Age in m + 9)/2 kg
Above 1 year	(Age + 3) × 2.2 kg

Height gain

Rate of height	Velocity
1st 3 months	3.5 cm/month
Next 3 months (4–6)	2 cm/month
Next 3 months(7–9)	1.5 cm/month
Next 3 months(10–12)	1.2 cm/month

Weech's formula

(age × 6) + 77 cm

Arm span: It is the distance between tips of middle fingers of both arms when the arms are outstretched at right angles to the body facing away from the wall.

Age	Arm spam
Below 5 years	2 cm < height
5–10 years	1 cm < height
At 10 years	Arm span = height
Above 10 years	Arm span > height by 2 cm

Note: Arm span > height – Marfan syndrome, Klinefelter's syndrome, homocystinuria.

Arm span < height – achondroplasia, cretinism.

Upper segment—lower segment ratio

At birth	1.7:1
At 6 months	1.6:1
At 1 year	1.5:1
At 2 years	1.4:1
At 3 years	1.3:1
At 4 years	1.2:1
At 5 years	1.1:1
7–10 years	1:1
Adult	1:1.1

Note: Proportionate short stature—US : LS ratio is normal for age
Disproportionate dwarfism—US : LS ratio is not normal for age.

Mid-arm circumference
(Age independent criteria between 1 and 5 years)

At birth	11–12 cm
At 1 year	15–16 cm

Arnold's classification

>13.5 cm	Normal
12.5–13.5 cm	Moderate PEM
<11.5 cm	Severe PEM

Shakir tape: plastic tape with colored zones—green, yellow and red

Green	13.5 cm
Yellow	12.5–13.5 cm
Red	<12.5 cm

Head circumference

At birth	33–35 cm	0–3 months	2 cm/month
3 months	39–41 cm		
6 months	42–44 cm	4–6 months	1 cm/month

Contd ...

Contd ...

1 year	45–47 cm		
3 years	47–49 cm	6–12 months	0.5 cm/month
5 years	49–51 cm	1–2 years	2 cm/year
7 years	50–51 cm		
12 years	51.5–53 cm	2 years	0.5 cm/year

Note: Dines formula—for estimating HC in 1st year of life—[(length in cm + 9.5) +/–2.5]/2

Microcephaly: Reduction in HC by more than 3 SD from normal.
Macrocephaly: Increase in HC by more than 2 SD from normal.
1 SD = 2.5% of value (approx. 1.25 cm)

Chest circumference

At birth	31 cm
HC = CC	1 year
After 1 year	CC > HC

Note: In malnourished case CC < HC even beyond 1 year

Grading of wasting based on weight for height

>90%	No wasting
80–90%	Mild
70–80%	Moderate
< 70%	Severe

Waterlow's grading of stunting based on height for age

>95%	Normal
90–95%	Grade I stunting
85–90%	Grade II stunting
<85%	Grade III stunting

	Weight	Height
Double	4 months	4 years
Triple	12 months	12 years

Developmental Assessment (Only in CP Cases)

- Ventral suspension supine position
- Supine to sitting neonatal reflexes

(According to the new examination pattern one can omit the dietetic history and need not do the anthropometric measurements in the clinical case. While in the nutrition case, one has to take the dietetic history, anthropometry and assess the nutritional status).

Nutrition Annexure

Item	Quantity	Kcal	Protein
Cooked rice	1 cup	175	4
Uncooked ragi	6 tsp	100	2
Dosa	1	70	2
Iddly	1	50	2
Chapati	1	70	2
Puri	1	35	1
Uppuma	1 cup	250	6
Bread	1 Slice	70	2
Pathiri	1	50	1
Porotta	1	100	3
Puttu	50	2	1
Biscuit	1	20	0.5
Vadai	1	50	1
Bonda	1	50	1
Ground nuts	10	20	1
Banana	1	100	1
Plantain	1	50	1
Egg	1	80	6
Mutton	1 oz	50	6
Beef	1 oz	30	6
Fish	1 oz	80	6
Sardine (methi)	1	30	3

Measures

1 tea spoon	5 mL
1 table spoon	15 mL
1 cup	200 mL
1 tumbler	250 mL

Expected Calories

ICMR recommendation

0–6 months	108 cal/kg
6 m–1 year	098 cal/kg
1, 2, 3 years	1240 cal
4, 5, 6 years	1690 cal
7, 8, 9 years	1950 cal
10, 11, 12 years	1970 cal (F) 2190 cal (M)
Adolescent	2100 cal (F) 2500 cal (M)

Item	Quantity	Kcal	Protein
Cows milk	100 mL	70	3.5
Human milk	100 mL	70	1.5
Volume at 6 months	600	700 mL	
Volume at 1 year	400	500 mL	
Pappad	1	20	0.5
Cooked dal	1 tsp	8	0.5
Smash potato	1 tsp	40	0
GLV	50 g	50	0
Upperi	1 help	10	0.5
Sambar	1 cup	50	2.5
Fruits	100 g	60	0.5
Coconut	100 g	444	4.5
Sugar/jaggery	1 tsp	20	0
Oils/ghee	I tsp	36	0

Working formula for calories (Bedside calculation)

At 1 year 1000 calories, after that add 100 months for every year.

Tip: It is seen that in spite of the child having adequate growth the calorie intake is pretty low and the protein usually adequate. This is due to faulty calculation. In these circumstances the coconut 1, 2, 3 years chutney will come to help (See the calorie of coconut). 1 cup of tea/ coffee containing half glass milk and 1 tsp sugar will give 90 cal and 3.5 g protein.

Expected Proteins

(IMCR recommendation)

0–6 months	2.05 gm/kg
6 m–1 year	1.65 gm/kg
1–3 years	22 gm
4–6 years	30 gm
7–9 years	41 gm
10–12 years	54 gm (M) 57 gm (F)
Adolescent	60 gm (F) 70 gm (M)

Newborn History Taking and Examination

History

- *General:* Mother's name and age, parity, last menstrual period, expected date of delivery
- *Past obstetric history:* Past pregnancies—when gestation, neonatal problems, present status.
- *Antenatal care:* Registration, contacts (when, number), where/by whom, tests (Hb, urine albumin/sugar, cultures, ultrasound, blood group, VDRL, HIV, others), TT immunization, diet, supplements (iron, folic acid, calcium, iodine).
- *Obstetric/Medical complications:* Obstetric complications (toxemia, UTI, twins/triplets, placenta previa, accidental hemorrhage); fetal problems (IUGR, hydrops, Rh isoimmunization); medical problems (diabetes, hypertension); investigations, medications, course.
- *Labor:* Presentation, lie, onset of labor (spontaneous/induced), rupture of membranes (spontaneous/artificial), liquor (clear/ meconium stained); duration of first and second stage of labor; fetal heart rate (tachycardia, bradycardia, irregular).

- *Delivery:* Place of delivery, conducted by whom, vaginal (spontaneous/forceps/vacuum), cesarian (indication, elective/emergency); local/general anesthesia; other drugs; duration of third stage; postpartum hemorrhage.
- *Immediate care at birth:* Resuscitation, time of first breath/cry, APGAR scores if known; cord care; passage of urine/stool.
- *Feeding history:* What feeds; breastfeeding (when initiated, frequency, adequacy); other feeds (what, how fed).
- *Postnatal problems:* Any problems experienced (feeding problems, jaundice, eye discharge, fever), their course/investigations/treatment; any problems at present.
- *Family history:* History of health problems in the family
- *Past medical problems:* History of past medical problems, if any
- *Personal/Social history:* Socioeconomic status, family support.

Examination

- *Immediately after birth:* Weight, gestation, congenital anomalies, sex assigning, APGAR scores, umbilical cord examination, examination of the placenta.

General

- *Appearance:* Overall appearance—well/sick look; alert/unconscious.
- *Vital signs*: Temperature, cold stress; respiratory rate, retractions, grunt/stridor; heart rate, palpable femorals; blood pressure, capillary refill time, cry.
- *Anthropometry:* Weight, length, head circumference, chest circumference
- *Gestation:* Assessment by physical criteria—more detailed assessment by New Ballard examination
- *Classification by intrauterine growth:* Appropriate/small/large for gestational age; symmetric/asymmetric small for gestational age; signs of IUGR (loose folds of skin, poor muscle mass, wrinkles over thighs/buttocks.
- *Congenital:* Head to toe examination for malformations/abnormalities.
- *Birth trauma:* Search for trauma; cephalhematoma.
- *Common signs:* Cyanosis, jaundice (extent), bleed, pustules, edema, pallor, bleeding, fontanel.
- *Special signs:* Caput, eye discharge, umbilical examination (stump, discharge, redness), development peculiarities (toxic erythema, ebstein pearls, breast engorgement, vaginal bleeding, capillary hemangiomas, Mongolian spot).

- *Feeding:* Observe feeding on breast (Check signs of positioning and attachment).
- *Reflexes:* Moro, grasp, rooting.

Systemic Examination

- *Chest:* Shape, distress, retractions, air entry, adventitious sounds
- *CVS:* Precordium, apical impulse, heart sounds/murmur.
- *Abdomen:* Distention, wall edema, tenderness, palpable liver/spleen/kidneys, any other lump, ascites, hernial sites, gonads, genitalia,
- *Musculoskeletal system:* Deformities, test for developmental dysplasia of hip, club foot.
- *Central nervous system:* State; cranial nerve examination (Vision, pupils, eye movement examination, facial sensation and motility, hearing, sucking and swallowing); motor examination (Tone and posture, power, tendon reflexes).

Inherited conditions screened for at birth

- Phenylketonuria
- Hypothyroidism
- Hemoglobinopathies in vulnerable groups
- Cystic fibrosis in affected families
- Congenital adrenal hyperplasia

Examination Tips

- Height/Length
  (Length—below 2 years—Infantometer)
  (Height—above 2 years—Stadiometer)
  - Make the child stand bare feet on a level floor
  - Feet slightly separated
  - Heels, buttocks and back are brought in contact with the wall
  - Head is so positioned so that the child looks directly forwards with the Frankfurt plane (Line joining floor of external auditory meatus to the floor of the orbit) and the biauricular plane horizontal
  - The head piece (Firm card board/long scale) is kept firmly over the vertex to compress the hair and mark the point using pencil
  - Remove the child

- The 0 of the tape is fixed at the floor and is measured upwards to the fixed drawn point
- Note the height. Compare it with the required weight if you have time.

- Weight
  (Most reliable criterion of assessment of the health and nutritional status of children)
  - Scale has an accuracy of +/- 20 gm (Beam type weighing scale)
  - Electronic weighing scale for infants (+/- 1 to 5 gm) and children (+/- 10 gm) are more accurate
  - *Bathroom type:* Scales are very unreliable
  - In field conditions, Salter spring scales are useful.
- Head circumference (HC)
  - Ideally use a fiber glass tape
  - Tape should encircle the most prominent part of the occiput and the supraorbital frontal area
  - The occipitofrontal head circumference is measured by the overlapping technique.
- Chest circumference (CC)
  - Keep the child in recumbent position
  - Measure at the level of the nipple, midway between expiration and inspiration.
  - It is ideal to note the CC during full inspiration and full expiration if chest expansion is also required like in a respiratory case.
    (*Note:* Normally, HC = CC at 9 months of age, but this is earlier in preterm babies and later in malnourished children.)
- Mid-arm circumference (MAC)
  - Measure using fiber glass or steel tape
  - Use the overlapping technique
  - With the child sitting or standing, semiflex his LEFT upper limb at the elbow and mark the midpoint between acromion and olecranon process.
  - Now, the child is made to keep his left upper limb by the side of his body and measure MAC at that level.
  - *Shakir tape:* A fiber glass tape with 3 colors (for use by field staff)
  - *Red:* <12.5 cm (Severe malnutrition)
  - *Yellow:* 12.5–13.5 cm (Moderate malnutrition)
  - *Green:* > 13.5 cm (No malnutrition)
  - *Bangle test:* Internal diameter 4 cm
  - If it passes above the elbow, it suggests that upper arm is <12.5 cm (severe malnutrition).

- *Quac stick:* Principle—acute starvation mainly affects MAC; height remains unaffected. The expected height of the child against various values of MAC are inscribed on the rod. If malnourished, the child would be taller than the anticipated height from the MAC.
- Thickness of subcutaneous fat with Heberden's calipers, measured over triceps or subscapular region.
- Fat thickness is >10 mm among healthy children between 1 to 6 years of age. Those <6 mm indicate severe malnutrition.

- Upper segment—lower segment ratio
  - *Upper segment:* From vertex to upper edge of symphysis pubis
  - *Lower segment:* From symphysis to heel
  - *Ideally US:* LS ratio is taken only if the height is grossly abnormal.
- Arm span
  - Ask the child to face the wall and place his chest and extended arms in contact with the chest wall.
  - Mark the tips of the middle fingers of both arms on the walls and ask the child to move away.
  - Now, measure the distance between these two points.
- Pallor
  - Take the child near the window for good vision.
  - Both palpebral conjunctiva should be inspected simultaneously, with slightly everting the lower eyelid (As undue stretch will drain the blood even in the normal person making it appear pale).
  - Inspect oral mucosa, hard palate, nailbed and palmar creases (pale when, Hb at 7 g%).
- Clubbing (in day light)
  - Hold the fingers at eye level and look for loss of onychodermal angle.
  - Feel for fluctuation at the nail base.
  - Look for clubbing in all the fingers of both upper limbs.
    Ask the patient to oppose the dorsal aspects of both thumbs and look for loss of rhomboid shape in between them.
  - Inspect the toe nails for clubbing.
  - Palpate firmly over the medial and lateral aspects of the wrists to rule any tenderness (in HPOA).
- Jaundice (day light)
  - Place your left hand on the patient's forehead and lift both upper eyelids simultaneously.
  - Ask the patient to look at a tingerheld down.
  - Inspect the soft palate and mucosa, nail bed.

- *NEVER use torch light for looking for pallor, jaundice, cyanosis. How to differentiate cyanosis of tongue from mucosal pigmentation (in day light).
    - Inspect other mucosal surfaces.
    - Try to blanch using a glass slide; cyanosis blanches, not pigmentation.
    - Feel for temperature of distal parts of limbs (To rule out peripheral cyanosis).
- Pedal edema
  - Expose both lower limbs.
  - Press above the medial malleolus on both sides simultaneously and hold for at least 30 seconds.
  - Look and palpate for any depression.
  - Find the upper level of the edema.

Cardiovascular System

Shift of Mediastinum

The child should be looking straight and should be at the same level as the examiner

- Look for trails sign
- Look for apex beat
  - Whether at the level of nipple or below
  - Whether medial or lateral to nipple
- Inspect the spine for kyphosis or scoliosis
- Palpate the trachea—place the index and ring finger over the medial end of both clavicles and run the middle finger over the trachea
- Make the child to lie down and inspect obliquely
- Palpate the apex beat starting from the midclavicular line using the palm, then the ulnar aspect of the hand and finally with the finger
- Find the midclavicular line and see if the apex beat is medial or lateral to the midclavicular line.

Palpation for Apex Beat

- Rule out any kyphosis or scoliosis
- Patient lying supine
- Inspect obliquely for any visible apical impulse using the palm of the hand, start palpating from the mid-axillary line

- Once an impulse is felt, use the ulnar border and finally localize with the index finger
- If apex cannot be localized in the supine position, make the patient sit up and then lean forward and in the left lateral position. Even if not palpable thus, palpate on the right side to rule out dextrocardia.

Palpation of Second Heart Sound

- Localize the apex beat
- Palpate the pulmonary area
- Palpate both apex and pulmonary area with palm simultaneously to find if it is the same sound.

Gastrointestinal System

Elicit Shifting Dullness

Child in supine position

- Percuss over the midline downwards till the bladder dullness is reached (Keep your finger horizontally).
- Keep fingers vertically, percuss from midline laterally till dullness is reached, continue percussing till it is completely dull and percuss back to the point, where the dullness started.
- Now, ask the patient to lie in the opposite lateral position, wait for 2 minutes and percuss from resonant to dull area.

Palpation of Liver

- Expose till mid-thigh (cover external genitalia)
- Patient lying down and examiner sitting on a stool
- Ask the child to flex his knee
- Ask the patient to turn his head to the opposite side and breathe deeply with mouth open
- Start palpating from the right iliac fossa upwards looking at the face of the patient for any tenderness
- Fingers should be para1lel to the upper border of the liver
- Feel the lower border of the liver touching the palpating finger
- Find the lower border of liver and measure how much the liver is enlarged in the midclavicular line
- Repeat the above procedure in the midline to find the enlargement of the left lobe of liver and measure enlargement below xiphisternum

- Percuss from above, downwards in the midclavicular costal tenderness (Percussion of the lower border of liver starting from right iliac fossa).
- Ask the patient to take deep inspiration and do tidal percussion (inference-mass is below the diaphragm)
- Find the liver span
- Auscultate over the mass (liver) for any rub or venous hum
- Pulsation of the liver—ask the patient to sit and place the hand in front and behind at the lower end of costal margin (enlarged liver) and ask the patient to hold his breath. Look for anteroposterior pulsation.

Description of liver enlargement

- Tender/nontender
- Uniform or one lobe enlarged
- Consistency
- Soft firm, hard
- Margin—sharp, rounded
- Surface—smooth, nodular (umbilicated, nonumbilicated)
  Note: Never comment about liver span in presence of right sided pleural effusion.

Palpation of Spleen

- Patient in supine position
- Start palpating from right iliac fossa obliquely upwards
- Fingers parallel to the left costal margin
  - Ask the patient to turn his head to the opposite side and breathe deeply with mouth open
  - Try to palpate the splenic notch and look for tenderness
  - Measure the enlargement of spleen from MCC on left costal margin along the axis of spleen
  - Percuss over the midaxillary line and see if the 5th space is dull. If yes, there is splenic enlargement
  - Auscultate for splenic rub and venous hum.

Nervous System

Test the Optic Nerve

Visual acuity

This should ideally be checked by using a Snellen's chart: (So mention that as the Snellen's chart was not available accurate measurement of visual acuity could not be made and only a rough assessment by finger counting could be made. Order of assessment—Visual acuity at 6 m—cannot read topmost line—Assess at 5-4-3-2-1 m-Finger counting at 1 m—Finger counting close to face—Hand movements—Projection of light—Light perception).

Color vision ideally requires an Ishihara's chart. So, only a rough assessment can be made.

Visual field assessment: Always check the visual acuity before doing the visual field assessment.

Confrontation method

The patient is asked to sit 1 m apart, eyes at the same level.

The child is asked to close his right eye and the examiner's left eye. And ask the child to look straight into the examiner's eye.

The hand should be held midway between the two and should be brought in an oblique line and ask the child to tell when he sees the finger first.

After checking the upper and lower quadrants on the same side, the examiner must close his right eye with his right hand (So that the right hand does not obstruct vision while crossing).

Now repeat the procedure in the opposite eye.

N.B.: Ask the child to close the eyes, in a cupped manner in order to prevent pressure on the eyes.

Check for visual inattention by a procedure similar to confrontation test. If the child can see finger movements when done unilaterally on both sides but can see only one side when both fingers are moved simultaneously. In CP cases and in unconscious patients, look for menace reflex using slicing action of the palm).

Test the IIIrd, IVth and VIth Cranial Nerves

- First ask the child to look into your eyes and fix his head using your left hand
- Look for ptosis, squint, nystagmus, shape, size and symmetry of pupil
- Check for saccadic movements by asking the child to look to the left, right, up and down
- Now check the pursuit movements, finger kept at about 20 to 30 cm from the child at the eye level
- Ask the child to follow the movements of the finger as it is moved
- As the finger reaches to one side (But still in the binocular field of vision)
  - Ask for diplopia
  - Look for nystagmus

- Repeat on the opposite side
- Now check for movements in all the 9 cardinal positions.
  (If the obliques are paralyzed, one can look for intorsion or extorsion by looking at one blood vessel in the sclera and looking for its movements).
- Check for light reflex both direct and indirect
  For better visualization of indirect reflex light a torch with a dim light on the side in such a way that it does not produce a light reflex on its own.
- Ask the child to place his hand on the center of face so that the other eye is protected from the light of the torch. The torch should be brought from side to the front of the eye
- Repeat the same procedure on the opposite eye
- Check for accommodation reflex.
  - Place the torch with dim light on the side of the eye.
  - Now ask the child to look far away and then to the finger placed on the tip of the finger.
  - Now ask to look again far away, at this moment the dilatation of the pupil which occurs is more easier to visualize than the constriction which occurs on looking the tip of the nose.
- In unconscious patient or a very small child look for Doll's eye movement which has two inferences:
  - The cortical control on brainstem is lost (As this reflex is inhibited in conscious individuals by the cortex)
  - The brainstem is intact.

Test for Vth Cranial Nerve

Motor part

- Ask the child to open his mouth against resistance of a fist placed below the jaw and look for deviation of the jaw
- If there is a simultaneous VIIth nerve palsy place, a scale between the two upper central incisor and look for deviation of the mandible
- Ask the child to clench his teeth and palpate the masseter and temporalis on both sides.

Sensory part

Check pain, touch and temperature in the area of supply of all three branches of Vth nerve. Remember that the sensory area of Vth extends on the scalp to a line joining the two ears (Like a headphone and on the bridge of the nose). The angle of the mandible is not a sensory area of Vth nerve (it is of cervical nerves C2, C3).

Reflexes

Superficial reflexes (Corneal and conjunctival reflexes).

Ask the child to look to the opposite side and bring a wisp of cotton from the side and touch the corneoconjunctival junction (or at the lateral aspect of the bulbar conjunctiva).

In children with long eyelashes, using your fingers slightly evert the lower eyelid so that the eyelashes do not come in contact with the cotton wisp which may also produce a blink (false +ve).

Never touch the center of the cornea as it may cause ulceration.

Always ask the child if they felt the sensation.

If the 7th nerve is paralyzed on the same side, look for blinking on the opposite side.

Deep reflex (Jaw jerk)

- Ask the child to slightly open the mouth
- Place your finger over the chin of the child
- Hit the finger slightly with a knee hammer in a vertically downward direction.

Test for VIIth Cranial Nerve

Inspection

- Ask the child to close his eyes tightly.
- If the child has LMN palsy, we can notice the Bell's phenomenon, but in UMN palsy, the child would have some weakness in closing his eyes but no Bell's phenomenon.
- Look for loss of nasolabial folds, deviation of the angle of the mouth to the opposite side, weakness of platysma, loss of wrinkling on the same side, drooling of saliva, difficulty to blow cheeks.

Palpation

- Fix the head of the child and ask him to follow the finger placed horizontally as it is raised upwards.
- Look for wrinkling of the forehead. There may be creases on forehead even when looking straight ahead which may not be lost even with facial nerve palsy. If in doubt ask the child to raise his eyebrows.
- Ask the child to close his eyes and the examiner must try to forcefully open it.
- Ask the child to blow his cheek and look for air escaping from the paralyzed side.
- Taste sensation on the anterior 2/3rd of the tongue (usually not done but is a favorite question).

- Tell the child to raise 1 finger if sweet and 2 fingers if salty and tell him not to withdraw the tongue.
- Ask the child to protrude his tongue, now hold his tongue with a swab and dry it. Now, drop a solution on one side and ask the child to indicate whether sweet or salty (Never allow the child to put the tongue back into the month).
- Wipe the tongue dry and repeat it on the opposite side.

Hyperacusis

- Place one earpiece of the stethoscope in one ear of the child and place the bar of the vibrating tuning fork over the diaphragm, the child will complain of very loud noise if hyperacusis is present.

Test for IXth and Xth Nerves

Inspection

- Position of the median raphe
- Position of the uvula (base)
- Simultaneous and symmetrical upward movement of the soft palate on saying 'Ah'.

Palpation

- Gag reflex—Use a tongue depressor and touch the posterior pharyngeal wall on each side and look for gag reflex.
- Ask the child if he feels the sensation.
  The swab for touching the posterior pharyngeal wall can be made by cutting one end or an ear bud and inserting a stick into the straw.
- Taste on the posterior 1/3rd of the tongue cannot be tested clinically.

Test for XIIth Cranial Nerve

Inspection

- When the tongue is placed in the floor of the mouth look for fasciculation and tremor
- Look for wasting of the tongue
- Ask the child to protrude the tongue and look for deviation
- Looking for food residue in the gap between the gums and cheek.

Palpation

Ask the child to push the tongue against the cheek and offer resistance.

Looking for Plantar Response

- Expose up to the thighs (To visualize the tensor fascia lata)
- Looking for the sensation on the sole

- Looking for the mobility of the big toe
- Fix the ankle and feet should be perpendicular to the bed
- Do not stroke the base of the big toe. The first movement of the big toe must be taken into account
- Repeat the same procedure on the opposite side
- If no response to one side and flexor response on the opposite side, the side with no response is taken as extensor.

Looking for Knee Jerk (Applicable to the Other Deep Tendon Jerks)

- Expose up to the thigh
- Check mobility of the joint
- Palpate the patellar tendon
- Look on the medial side of the thigh while hitting the tendon by a swinging action of the knee hammer.

If no response, repeat the procedure by reinforcement (Clenching of the teeth at the point of contact between the hammer and the tendon. If still not obtained knee jerk is taken as absent).

Never hold the contracting muscles while testing the jerks.

Looking for Cerebellar Signs

Finger nose test: Ask the child to reach out for the finger thus testing the intentional tremor which is clearly seen at the terminal part of this movement.

Heel knee test: The child should slide his heel (and not the gap between the heel and the lateral malleoli) from knee over the shin to the big toe, then keep it by the side and again place the heel on the knee and repeat it. Repeat it on the opposite side.

Rebound phenomenon (Protect the eyes of the child using the palm)

Pendular knee jerk (more than 2.5 movements).

Looking for Signs of Meningeal Irritation

Neck rigidity

First turn the head to both sides to rule out other bony causes and then using four fingers of both hands and the thumbs at the forehead flex the neck. (Simultaneously look for the flexion of tile hips suggestive of positive Brudzinski's neck sign).

Kernig's sign

Flex the hip at 90° and then extend the knee and look for any restriction of the movement due to spasm of hamstrings and also pain.

Simultaneously, look for flexion of the other knee suggestive positive Brudzinski's leg sign).

Brudzinski's sign

Fundoscopy (not done).

MISCELLANEOUS

Measurement of Temperature

Axillary temperature is taken in children less than 6 years (or older children who are not well oriented or mentally retarded).

If oral temperature is being taken, tell the patient that it is not at all painful and should not bite it.

- Take the thermometer and wipe it with a clean wisp of cotton see the mercury level
- Shake it to see if the level has fallen down
- Place the thermometer in the axilla or the oral cavity for ideally 3 minutes or a minimum of 1 minute
- Take the thermometer without touching the bulb
- Place the thermometer at the eyelevel and visualize it with a white background (and not the window) and take the reading

  For every 1°F rise of temperature:
  - Pulse increases by 10 beats per minute
  - Respiratory rate increases by 7/minute
  - BMR increases by 4

  For every 1°C
  - Pulse increases by 18 beats per minute
  - Oral temperature + 0.5° = Rectal temperature
  - Oral temperature - 0.5° = Axillary temperature
  - Normal body temperature 36.6°C - 7.2°C
  - Hypothermia < 35°C
  - Hyperpyrexia >41.6°C

Neonatal Reflexes

Rooting Reflex

- Stimulation of the infant's cheek near the angle of the mouth, the child seeks the finger.
- *Appears:* 32 weeks.
- After 1 month becomes less prominent disappears by 3 months.

Sucking Reflex

- Stimulation of the upper or lower lips, produces movement of the lips and tongue in the direction of the stimulus.
- *Appears:* 32 weeks. *Disappears:* As in rooting.

Grasp Reflex

- Baby's palm is stroked with the examiner's index finger; the baby's finger grasps it. The grasp is so strong that the whole weight of the body can be supported with this traction response.
- *Appears:* 28 weeks. *Disappears:* 2 to 3 months.

Moro's Reflex

- The baby is placed on a soft cot
- The procedure is explained to the mother
- The head is held using both the hands, flexed to 30°C and is dropped suddenly into the hands.

Positive Response

- Abduction of arm at shoulder
- Extension of arm at the elbow
- Opening up of the hand
- Adduction of the arms
- Flexion of the forearm.

Asymmetrical Response

- Erb's palsy
- Spastic hemiplegia
- Fracture humerus or fracture clavicle
- *Appears:* 28 to 32 weeks
- *Disappears:* 5 to 6 months

Glabellar Tap

- Gently tap at the glabella
- Both the eyelids of the neonate blinks.

Asymmetric Tonic Neck Reflex

- Infant supine
- Infant's head is turned suddenly to one side

- The arms and leg on the same side is extended while the opposite side goes into flexion
- If persisting more than 6 to 9 months suspect CP
- *Appears:* 35 weeks
- *Disappears:* 6 to 7 months.

Crossed Extension

When the foot is stroked over the leg held in extension on one side there is rapid flexion, adduction, extension of the opposite leg.

7 ENT Case Format

ENT CASE TAKING FORMAT

Name	
Age	
Sex	
Address	
Occupation	

Presenting Complaints (See symptoms)

- History of present illness
- Past history
- Personal history
- Family history
- Socioeconomic status
- Examination
  - General examination
  - Vitals.

EXAMINATION OF ENT

EAR

Symptoms

- Hearing loss/hard of hearing
- Ear ache
- Ear discharge
- Itching in the ear
- Tinnitus
- Dizziness/vertigo.

History

- Onset
- Duration
- Progression
- Severity
- Associated symptoms.

Examination

Right Left

- Pinna
- Preauricular area
- Postauricular area
- External auditory canal
- Tympanic membrane
  - Color
  - Position
  - Surface
  - Mobility
- Mastoid
  - Eustachian tube—Valsalva maneuver
  - Facial nerve function.

Functional Testing

- Voice test/paper test/watch test
- Tuning fork tests
  - Rinne test
  - Weber test
  - Schwabach test
  - ABC
- Vestibular function
- Nystagmus
- Fistula test
- Positional test.

Nose, Nasopharynx and Paranasal Sinuses

Symptoms

- Nasal obstruction/nasal discharge
- Epistaxis

- Postnasal drip
- Sneezing
- Snoring
- Change in voice
- Disturbance of smell
- Headache.

Examination

- External framework
- Vestibule
- Anterior rhinoscopy with thudicum nasal speculum
  - Nasal passage
  - Septum
  - Floor
  - Roof
  - Lateral wall
- Posterior rhinoscopy.

Functional Examination

- Cold spatula test
- Olfactory nerve function.

Paranasal Sinuses

- Maxillary sinus
- Frontal sinus
- Ethmoid sinus
- Sphenoid sinus.

Oral Cavity and Oropharynx

Symptoms

- Pain
- Disturbance of salivation and taste
- Trismus
- Lesions.

Examination

- Lips
- Buccal mucosa

- Gums and teeth
- Hard palate
- Tongue
- Floor of mouth
- Retromolar trigone
- Tonsils
- Anterior pillar
- Posterior pillar
- Soft palate
- Posterior pharyngeal wall
- Base of tongue and valleculae.

Larynx and Laryngopharynx

Symptoms

- Hoarseness of voice
- Respiratory obstruction
- Repeated clearing of throat
- Dysphagia
- Mass in neck
- Cough and expectoration.

Examination

- External examination
- Indirect laryngoscopy.

Neck

Cervical lymph nodes.

Other Systems

- Cardiovascular system
- Respiratory system
- Gastrointestinal system
- Nervous system.

Summary

Diagnosis

8 Ophthalmology Case Format

OPHTHALMOLOGY CASE TAKING FORMAT

Name	
Age	
Sex	
Address	
Occupation	

Presenting Complaints

- Defective vision
- Watering/discharge
- Redness
- Asthenopic symptoms
- Photophobia
- Foreign body sensation
- Burning/itching sensation
- Pain
- Deviation of eye
- Diplopia
- Black spots in front of eyes
- Colored halos
- Distorted vision.

History of Present Illness

- Past history
- Personal history
- Family history
- Socioeconomic status
- Examination
- General examination
- Vitals.

Ocular Examination

	Right	Left
• Visual acuity		
• Visual field		

External Ocular Examination

- Head posture
- Forehead
- Eyebrows.

Eyelids

- Position
- Movements
- Lid margin
- Skin
- Palpebral aperture.

Lacrimal Apparatus

- Sac
- Puncta
- Regurgitation test.

Eyeball

- Position
- Visual axis
- Size
- Movements—six cardinal directions.

Conjunctiva

- Bulbar conjunctiva
- Lower palpebral conjunctiva and lower fornix
- Upper palpebral conjunctiva
- Superior fornix.

Discoloration/congestion/chemosis/follicles/papillae/foreign bodies/scarring/pinguecula/pterygium

Sclera

- Discoloration
- Inflammation
- Staphyloma
- Traumatic perforations.

Cornea

- Size
- Shape
- Surface
- Sheen
- Transparency
- Vascularization
- Corneal sensations.

Iris

- Color
- Synechiae
- Coloboma.

Pupil

- Number
- Location
- Size
- Shape
- Color
- Pupillary reaction
  - Direct light reflex
  - Consensual light reflex
  - Swinging flash light test
  - Near reflex.

Lens

- Position
- Shape
- Color
- Transparency.

IOP-digital Tonometry

Other Systems

- Cardiovascular system
- Respiratory system
- Gastrointestinal system
- Nervous system.

Summary

Diagnosis

Index

O

P

Q

R

S

T

U

V

W